Skin disorders

YOUR QUESTIONS ANSWERED

KT-146-908

WITHDRAWN

For Elsevier

Commissioning Editor: Fiona Conn
Project Development Manager: Isobel Black
Project Manager: Nancy Arnott
Design Direction: George Ajayi
Illustration Manager: Bruce Hogarth
Illustrator: Chartwell

Skin disorders

YOUR QUESTIONS ANSWERED

Tim Mitchell
MBChB MRCGP DRCOG DPD
General Practitioner
Montpelier Health Centre
Bristol, UK

Cameron Kennedy
MA MB BChir FRCP
Consultant Dermatologist at Bristol Royal
Infirmary, Bristol Royal Hospital for
Children and Southmead Hospital,
Bristol, UK

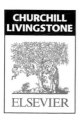

CHURCHILL
LIVINGSTONE

ELSEVIER

EDINBURGH LONDON NEW YORK OXFORD PHILADELPHIA ST LOUIS SYDNEY TORONTO 2006

CHURCHILL
LIVINGSTONE
ELSEVIER

First published 2006

ISBN 0 4430 7463 1

British Library Cataloguing in Publication Data
A catalogue record for this book is available from the British Library

Library of Congress Cataloging in Publication Data
A catalog record for this book is available from the Library of Congress

Note
Knowledge and best practice in this field are constantly changing. As new research and experience broaden our knowledge, changes in practice, treatment and drug therapy may become necessary or appropriate. Readers are advised to check the most current information provided (i) on procedures featured or (ii) by the manufacturer of each product to be administered, to verify the recommended dose or formula, the method and duration of administration, and contraindications. It is the responsibility of the practitioner, relying on their own experience and knowledge of the patient, to make diagnoses, to determine dosages and the best treatment for each individual patient, and to take all appropriate safety precautions. To the fullest extent of the law, neither the publisher nor the authors assume any liability for any injury and/or damage to persons or property arising out of or related to any use of the material contained in this book.

The Publisher

Working together to grow
libraries in developing countries

www.elsevier.com | www.bookaid.org | www.sabre.org

ELSEVIER   BOOK AID
International   Sabre Foundation

The
publisher's
policy is to use
paper manufactured
from sustainable forests

Printed in China

Contents

Preface

Skin disease is very common – it accounts for up to 20% of consultations with GPs in the UK. This is not all that surprising as the skin is the largest organ in the body and there are in excess of 2000 different diseases. It is fortunate, therefore, that the majority of skin problems presenting in primary care fit into one of nine categories.

On the face of it, it would seem logical to assume that GPs would start their professional lives well equipped to deal with basic skin problems and rapidly gain greater experience and expertise. That this is not usually the case is largely due to the lack of any statutory requirement for GPs to learn any dermatology as part of their training. It is not just GPs, as the work done by the All Party Parliamentary Group on Skin shows, who suffer from a lack of training. None of the standard professional groups involved in primary medical care has to be trained in dermatology before they are licensed to practise. This includes nurses, health visitors, midwives and pharmacists. It is to be hoped that this situation will change in the UK in the near future as our secondary care services cannot cope with an ever-increasing workload.

Skin disease is not just a 'cosmetic nuisance'; it can have a profound impact on a patient's life. This impact does not necessarily correlate with the extent and severity of the disease and this must be remembered when managing a patient. It can be helpful to think of five 'Ds' in association with dermatology:

- Disfigurement
- Discomfort
- Disability
- Depression
- Death.

This book cannot claim to be a comprehensive guide to treating skin disease in primary care as, unlike others in the series, it does not have the luxury of concentrating on one disease. It will answer some of the common questions relating to the most prevalent diseases but can only do this by assuming that the reader has some diagnostic ability and is willing to read further to gain a more in-depth insight.

How to use this book

The *Your Questions Answered* series aims to meet the information needs of GPs and other primary care professionals who care for patients with chronic conditions. It is designed to help them work with patients and their families, providing effective, evidence-based care and management.

The books are in an accessible question and answer format, with detailed contents lists at the beginning of every chapter and a complete index to help find specific information.

ICONS

Icons are used in the book to identify particular types of information:

 highlights information important to clinical practice

 highlights side-effect information.

PATIENT QUESTIONS

At the end of relevant chapters there are sections of frequently asked patient questions, with easy-to-understand answers aimed at the non-medical reader. These questions are also listed at the end of the book.

A background to skin disease

1

1.1 What is the structure of the skin?

The skin is the largest organ in the body and is not simply a layer of cells holding the body together. It has a surface area of 1.8 m² and makes up about 16% of body weight. It is made up of three layers – the epidermis, the dermis and the subcutis (*Fig. 1.1*).

The epidermis is the outer layer made up of keratinocytes, in various stages of maturation, melanocytes and Langerhans cells (*Box 1.1*). It is usually about 0.1 mm thick but is much thicker on the palms and soles – up to 1.4 mm.

The dermis is a tough matrix of supportive connective tissue containing specialized structures. It too varies in thickness – from 0.6 mm on the eyelids to 3 mm or more on the palms, soles and back. It is made up of collagen for strength, elastin for elasticity and a ground substance which is a semi-solid matrix. The main cells are fibroblasts, dendrocytes, mast cells, macrophages and lymphocytes.

The subcutis is made up of loose connective tissue and fat and can be up to 3 cm thick, especially over the abdomen.

1.2 What other structures are in the skin?

Hair is found over all the skin apart from in what is called 'glabrous skin' on the palms, soles, glans penis and introitus. It is divided into three types:

■ Lanugo – fine and long which grows on the fetus from 20 weeks and is usually shed before birth
■ Vellus – short fine hairs over most of the body surface

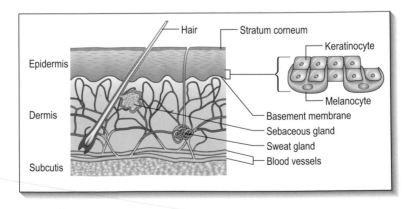

▲
Fig. 1.1 Structure of the skin.

BOX 1.1 Structure of the skin

Basal layer	Contains keratinocytes which are either dividing or not. They are secured to the basement membrane which separates the epidermis from the dermis. 5–10% of the cells are melanocytes which synthesize melanin and transfer it to the keratinocytes
Prickle cell layer	After division, the new keratinocytes move up from the basal layer to form an interconnected layer of polyhedral cells. Langerhans cells (dendritic, immunologically active cells) are mostly found in this layer
Granular cell layer	The keratinocytes become flattened and lose their nuclei. They contain granules which produce the lipid-rich intercellular glue
Horny layer	The outer layer consists of sheets of flattened, overlapping polyhedral cells now referred to as corneocytes. They are several cells thick on palms and soles but less thick elsewhere

---

- ■ Terminal – longer, thicker hairs which differentiate from vellus hairs after puberty with the influence of androgens. Found on the scalp, eyebrows, eyelashes, beard area, pubis and axillae.

Nail is a plate of hardened keratin which provides protection and helps with fine touch sensitivity.

Sweat glands are in the dermis and produce a watery secretion. Two types are identified:

- ■ Eccrine – 2.5 million are present all over the skin surface, most densely on the palms, soles, axillae and forehead
- ■ Apocrine – mainly around the axillae, perineum and areolae. They are remnants of mammalian sexual scent glands but produce an odourless secretion. The smell comes from bacterial action on the sweat.

The skin has a rich nerve supply, especially on the hands, face and genitalia. It also contains many blood and lymphatic vessels.

1.3 Does the skin have many different functions?

Yes. It is the last line of defence against the outside world, protecting our bodies from external attack and keeping the right conditions inside through its prevention of loss of fluid and regulation of temperature. It also allows for a display of individuality through decoration, jewellery and hair styling (*Box 1.2*).

BOX 1.2 Functions of the skin

- A barrier to physical agents including UV radiation
- Protection from mechanical injury
- Defence against microbes
- Homeostasis – prevents loss of water and electrolytes
- Regulates temperature and insulates
- Sensory functions
- Fine touch and grip
- Vitamin D synthesis
- Calorie store – subcutaneous fat
- Cosmetic, psychosocial and display functions

1.4 How common is skin disease?

This is quite difficult to answer as some studies show that only 25% of people with a skin problem consult a doctor. A community-based study in the UK showed that 22.5% of the population had a skin disease for which medical attention was thought to be necessary. A similar study in the USA put the figure at 31.2%. One study looking at use of medication in the UK found that 14% of adults and 19% of children had used a skin medication in the week prior to being questioned. Only 10% of the medication used had been obtained after receiving a prescription from a doctor.

1.5 Do skin diseases cause real problems for patients?

Yes, they do. Many skin diseases are chronic and relapsing and can produce a surprising amount of disability. Various quality of life studies have looked at the commonest chronic skin diseases such as eczema, psoriasis and acne, and shown that they can produce disability levels similar to:

- angina
- arthritis
- asthma
- back pain
- chronic bronchitis
- diabetes
- hypertension.

One of the leading lights of the Skin Care Campaign (*see Appendix*) suffers from psoriasis but also has coronary heart disease and diabetes. He has stated publicly that, if he were magically allowed to lose one of those three for ever, it would be the psoriasis. The main reason may be a sense of control over the heart disease and diabetes which is lacking for his psoriasis.

1.6   What are the commonest skin diseases?

 It is easier to answer this by listing categories of skin disease rather than individual diseases. There are nine categories which together account for some 70% of consultations in primary and secondary care in the UK for skin disease (*Fig. 1.2*):

- Skin cancer
- Acne
- Atopic eczema
- Psoriasis
- Viral warts
- Other infective skin disorders
- Benign tumours and vascular lesions
- Leg ulcers
- Contact dermatitis and other forms of eczema.

1.7   How should patients presenting with skin problems be assessed?

Taking a good history is the first and, probably, most important step. It is all too easy to rush straight into looking at a rash, especially if it is on exposed skin. There are many clues to be found in a thorough history taken

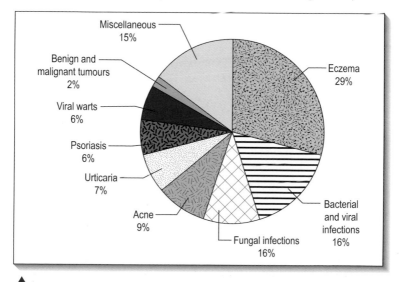

Fig. 1.2 Types of skin disease commonly seen in UK general practice.

after giving the patient a chance to talk about the problem in their own words (*Box 1.3*).

1.8 How should rashes be described and recorded in the notes?

It is very important to examine a patient with skin disease as fully as possible and in a good light. Resist the temptation to examine only the bit of skin presented by the patient. Ideally, the whole of the skin needs to be examined and the more widespread or unusual the rash, the more essential is a full examination. A correct diagnosis takes into account the distribution of the lesions, their morphology and configuration. If it is localized, note the absence of rash elsewhere; if it is widespread, look for symmetry and distinguish between a peripheral or central pattern. Check to see if only sun-exposed areas are affected, with sparing where the skin is shielded such as under the nose and chin. Involvement of flexures or extensor surfaces can give clues to likely diagnoses (e.g. atopic eczema in flexures, psoriasis on

---

BOX 1.3 Assessing patients with skin problems

■ History of the presenting problem
— How long has it been there?
— What did it look like at first?
— Has it changed – spread, sites affected, type of rash?
— Any symptoms – itch, burning, pain?
— Does anything make it worse, e.g. sunlight?
■ General health
— Any fever or other symptoms?
— Any other illnesses?
■ Past history
— Any previous skin problems?
— Any significant past illnesses, especially asthma and hay fever?
■ Family history
— Any skin problems or other chronic diseases?
■ Occupational and social history
— Type of employment?
— Any variation of the skin problem when not at work?
— Any hobbies?
— Any recent foreign travel?
— Alcohol and smoking?
■ Drug history
— Any regularly taken medication, whether prescribed or purchased?
— Anything used to treat this current rash?

extensor surfaces). It is also worth checking for any lesions the patient might not have noticed such as a small skin cancer on the back. The scalp, hair, nails, and inside the mouth should also be examined for any abnormalities.

Once the distribution has been noted, look at the morphology of individual lesions. *Table 1.1* shows a standard way of describing individual lesions which allows others to correctly interpret your findings.

Finally, the configuration of lesions should be looked at, noting such patterns as discrete, confluent, linear, grouped, annular or dermatomal.

1.9   What about scale and crusts and other changes in the skin?

Scale and crusts can be looked upon as secondary changes as they tend to arise from the primary lesions mentioned above or are the result of scratching.

- ■ *Scale* – this is an easily detached piece of the horny layer of the skin. Scale differs in thickness depending on the underlying condition but generally indicates an inflammatory process affecting the epidermis.
- ■ *Crust* – this might look like a scale but is made up of some sort of exudate which has dried – either blood or serous fluid.

Other common changes seen in the skin are:

- ■ *Atrophy*   this is a thinning of the skin and can represent changes in the epidermis, dermis or subcutaneous fat.
- ■ *Erosion* – this is caused by partial or complete loss of just the epidermis. Unlike ulcers, erosions heal without scarring.
- ■ *Excoriation* – this is the term used when an ulcer or an erosion has been caused by scratching.

TABLE 1.1   Standard descriptions of skin lesions

Type of lesion	Small (<0.5 cm)	Large (>0.5 cm)
Raised solid lesion	Papule	Plaque – if thin Nodule if also greater than 0.5 cm in depth
Flat area or different colour or texture	Macule	Large macule or patch
Fluid-filled raised lesion	Vesicle	Bulla
Pus-filled lesion	Pustule	Abscess
Leakage of blood into the skin	Petechiae (pinhead size) Purpura (up to 2 mm)	Ecchymosis Haematoma
Collection of oedema in the dermis	Weal	Weal – thin Angioedema – thicker and deeper

- *Fissure* – this is a split in the skin which usually extends through the epidermis into the upper layer of the dermis.
- *Lichenification* – this is the term given to skin which has become thickened, often from chronic rubbing or scratching. More prominent skin surface markings are evident.
- *Pigmentation* – this can be hyper- or hypo-, and often occurs after primary lesions heal.
- *Scar* – this can be used to describe any permanent change in the skin after damage but strictly speaking occurs when healing replaces normal skin structure with fibrous tissue.
- *Stria* – this is a linear area of atrophy from changes in the connective tissue. It can vary from white to purple in colour.
- *Telangiectasia* – dilated superficial blood vessel.
- *Ulcer* – this represents loss of the full thickness of epidermis and at least some of the dermis. Some ulcers extend right down into the fat layer.

Eczema

2

2.1   What is eczema?

The term eczema is used for a group of conditions which show a similar histology and to a lesser extent clinical appearances. The word eczema comes from the Greek and means to boil over. Vesicles are seen in some types of eczema (e.g. pompholyx, allergic contact and atopic eczema) if the inflammation is sufficiently intense, which is usually in the acute stage of the natural history. This may be over before the patient presents so is worth asking about when the history is taken. Even if there are no blisters, a histological section of eczema shows fluid between the keratinocytes, tending to push them apart. This oedema within the epidermis produces an appearance reminiscent of a sponge – hence the term spongiosis for the typical histological appearance. All the different conditions called eczema would be expected to show epidermal spongiosis, together with some degree of inflammation around superficial blood vessels.

2.2   Is eczema the same as dermatitis?

Yes, and no. Dermatitis is a broader concept, simply meaning inflammation of the skin. All eczema is dermatitis, but many conditions within the grouping dermatitis are not eczema (e.g. dermatitis herpetiformis). Most of the different types of eczema can, and often are, interchangeably termed dermatitis. More in the past than now, if an eczematous process was due to an irritant or allergic exposure at the workplace, it was designated contact dermatitis, and issues concerning compensation might at least have been implied. It is generally better to avoid such minefields and use the term eczema for such situations.

Partly because the clinical signs may be minimal (e.g. just itchy dry skin), many dermatologists use the term dermatitis instead of eczema for the cutaneous manifestations of atopy (excluding urticaria) but it is equally acceptable to name the condition atopic eczema.

For some of the eczemas, however, it is more commonplace to use 'dermatitis' (e.g. napkin (diaper) dermatitis, photodermatitis and neurodermatitis); for others, 'eczema' has been the preferred term (e.g. asteatotic eczema). For some of the rest (e.g. seborrhoeic, discoid (nummular) and gravitational), eczema and dermatitis are used interchangeably. The situation is, therefore, still very confusing and it is always worth finding out what terms are used most commonly in the area where you work and making sure that the terms you use are correctly understood by the patient.

2.3   Is there a simple way of classifying eczema?

Unfortunately, no. There are many recognizable triggers or causes for eczema: some are from the outside world (e.g. irritants, allergy and bacterial infection); others relate to the person with the eczema – for example, having a genetic tendency to eczema, asthma and hay fever, raised pressure in leg veins, and reacting to stressful circumstances. These trigger factors are independent of each other, so sometimes several can be important. Having looked carefully at all the circumstances, there are still some people in whom we do not know why the eczema is occurring. In these cases it is often still possible to classify the eczema in a descriptive sense, and there will be some knowledge about how it is best treated on the basis of previous similar patients.

As well as trying to give an appropriate label to the type of eczema, it is often useful with regard to therapy to classify the eczema in terms of time course and intensity of the process: *acute* means there has been a rapid onset and a short but perhaps severe course; *chronic* means continuing for a long time (*see Q 2.7*). This time course may give some extra clues as to the trigger(s) involved.

Our classification is, therefore, imperfect but designed to guide helpful investigation and treatment (*Table 2.1*).

2.4   What are the characteristic presentations of the different types of eczema?

Atopic
Atopy refers to a group of conditions (eczema, asthma and hay fever) where there is a very raised production of IgE in response to allergens in the environment. Seventy-five per cent of cases present before the age of 6 months, rising to 90% before the age of 5 years. It is thought to affect 20% of infants and 60–70% of affected children will have gone into remission by their early teenage years although they remain vulnerable to relapse. A general dryness of the skin may persist throughout life with the eczema varying in presentation with age.

■ In infancy it often starts on the face with vesicles and weeping. Distribution elsewhere is non-specific but it does tend to spare the napkin area.
■ As the child ages the distribution becomes more flexural around knees, elbows, wrists and ankles. The skin becomes increasingly thickened, dry and excoriated – often looking 'leathery'.
■ This pattern continues into adulthood with increasing lichenification and an increasing tendency to affect the trunk, face and hands.

Children with atopic eczema have intense itching and often scratch violently. Their sleep is badly affected and they may become hyperactive and manipulative, giving their parents a difficult time. Having one affected child can disrupt the life of a whole family.

Seborrhoeic

There are three different presentations which often merge together. Mainly hairy areas are affected with typical greasy yellowish scales in addition to the findings listed below. It may affect infants but is most common in adult males. The course is unpredictable and often chronic. A particularly severe form may present in patients with AIDS.

- A red, scaly rash on the scalp, ears, around the nose and nasolabial folds and eyebrows. It is often associated with otitis externa and blepharitis and causes 'cradle cap' in infants.
- On the trunk in the presternal and interscapular areas. Dry, scaly petaloid lesions sometimes accompanied by a more extensive outbreak of follicular papules and pustules.
- An intertriginous form affecting the axillae, umbilicus and groins which can also present under spectacles or hearing aids.

Discoid

The precise cause of this has yet to be identified but chronic stress may play a part. Infection with staphylococci and the release of bacterial antigens is also suspected to be a trigger. Lesions present typically on the limbs of middle-aged men, favouring the extensor surfaces, and are very itchy plaques, 5 cm or less in diameter. They show vesiculation and crusting and persist for many months, often recurring at the same sites.

Irritant contact

This is the commonest form of contact eczema – perhaps making up 80% of cases. Strong irritants will cause an obvious and acute reaction but weaker irritants need months or years of exposure to cause the same problems. The eczema usually affects the hands and forearms as the most common parts of the body exposed to detergents, industrial oils, solvents, etc. Many people with dry or fair skin are likely to develop irritant problems but a history of atopic eczema doubles the risk. Children can also get irritant eczema from bubble bath, modelling clays or dough and from constant lip-licking. The latter gives rise to a red, dry, fissured eczema around the mouth called 'lip-licking dermatitis'.

Allergic contact

This is a delayed hypersensitivity reaction (type IV) so behaves as follows:

- Previous contact is necessary to induce the response
- Response is specific to one substance
- All areas of skin will react once sensitization has taken place
- Sensitization often persists indefinitely and desensitization is unlikely to be possible.

TABLE 2.1 Eczema – a classification

Cause	Type of eczema	Trigger factor
Mainly caused by external triggers	Irritant	Chemicals, e.g. detergents Physical factors, e.g. friction
	Allergic	The immune system reacting – can often be tested
	Photodermatitis	Sunlight or artificial UV are necessary
Other types	Atopic	Often associated with hay fever, asthma and food allergies Flare ups common with irritants and skin infection
	Seborrhoeic	Essentially diagnosed by where it occurs and the appearance Skin surface yeasts important
	Venous (varicose, gravitational)	On the lower leg, due to high pressure in the veins, which are sometimes varicose
	Asteatotic	Crazy paving-like appearance, usually on the legs of the elderly, due to drying of the skin, e.g. from overwashing, a low humidity environment
	Pompholyx	Eruption of blisters on the fingers and toes, palms and soles
	Neurodermatitis	Also called lichen simplex – one or more itchy thickened sometimes lumpy patches or bumps, the result of repeated rubbing or scratching
	Discoid (nummular)	A descriptive term for rounded patches of eczema with no definable cause

2.5   Are there different patterns of presentation?

Various patterns are seen, depending on the original site of contact. Typical patterns might be nickel allergy under jewellery, watch straps and jeans studs; fingertip eczema from garlic; face and neck from perfume. An allergic cause should be suspected if the pattern of eczema is unusual (e.g. eyelids, around leg ulcers, hands or feet), there is known exposure to some of the common allergens, or the type of work is 'high risk' (e.g. hairdressing, nursing, gardening or floristry).

Asteatotic

This form of eczema occurs in old age. Patients may always have had a tendency to suffer dry skin made worse by low humidity in centrally heated rooms and the removal of natural oils from washing with soap. Diuretics can increase the problem from dehydration and hypothyroidism should be excluded. Asteatotic eczema presents on the legs which itch and show a background of dry skin with a superficial network of fine red lines, giving a 'crazy paving' appearance. These fine lines are actually fissures in the skin.

Venous

Also known as 'stasis' or 'gravitational', this is almost always linked to obvious venous insufficiency. The lower legs show chronic eczematous changes with pigmentation changes from haemosiderin deposition. Varicose veins and oedema may also be present. There is often an added element of contact allergic eczema as patients become sensitized to locally applied creams, especially topical antibiotics, or the preservatives in bandages. Ulceration may develop easily after excoriation.

Pompholyx

The cause of this is often unknown but it is linked to heat and emotional stress. Patients with nickel allergy may also develop pompholyx in response to low levels of nickel in foods. It is very itchy with recurring outbreaks of tense, thick-walled vesicles or larger blisters on the palms, along the fingers and sometimes on the soles. Each outbreak can last a few weeks and recur at irregular intervals.

Juvenile plantar dermatosis

This is thought to be linked to atopy so merits inclusion here. It is probably related to impermeability of modern materials and fabric used for socks and shoe linings. This leads to sweat gland blockage and a dry shiny eruption over the weight-bearing parts of the forefeet and toes. This can be accompanied by deep and painful fissures. No rash is seen in the toe webs so fungal infection is not a factor. It presents at any time after shoes first start to be worn and tends to clear spontaneously in the early teens.

Napkin dermatitis

This is probably the most common type of 'nappy rash' and is irritant in origin from the enzymes and ammonia released by urea-splitting bacteria. It is often complicated by Candida infection. The rash is a moist, sore erythema with a glazed appearance affecting the napkin area but sparing the skin folds (in contrast to seborrhoeic eczema). If Candida infection is present, 'satellite' lesions (erythematous papules or pustules) are seen around the periphery of the rash.

2.6 Are some types of eczema more common at different ages?

The age of onset can be helpful in deciding what type(s) of eczema a person has.

- Eczema in an infant is most commonly atopic (although this may appear discoid in places and can be aggravated by irritants) or seborrhoeic.
- In the child and teenager, atopic eczema is the commonest, but there will be some instances of contact allergy (e.g. to nickel).
- In adults of working age, irritant, contact allergic, seborrhoeic, discoid and atopic eczema are all common and can occur at many body sites; pompholyx and venous eczema are recognizable by their locations.
- The elderly are prone to asteatotic eczema, especially on the shins, and chronic idiopathic photodermatitis in addition to the types experienced by younger adults.

2.7 Does eczema look the same in acute and chronic stages?

Acute eczema will occur quite quickly – from hours to a few days – sometimes in previously normal skin. Vesicles may appear and then break to give a weeping surface. The underlying skin will be red, perhaps swollen, and often a little bumpy. Most acute eczema is very itchy; when the skin surface has broken down, this may be replaced by soreness. As days go by, crusting and then scaling may occur alongside the weeping or gradually replace it (*Fig. 2.1*).

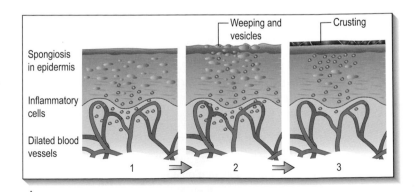

▲
Fig. 2.1 Progression of acute eczema.

Chronic eczema means it has been present for a long time – usually weeks at least. The ongoing inflammation, rubbing and scratching all contribute to an increased thickness of the skin (*Fig. 2.2*), which may develop a leathery appearance and show much more prominent skin surface markings. In dark skin, there may be changes in the pigmentation – both an increase and a decrease are possible. This thickened skin is liable to split, producing painful fissures, especially over the joints, palms and soles.

2.8 What other diseases could be confused with eczema?

Because of the wide range of appearances of eczema – for example depending on the type, body site and whether acute or chronic – there are several conditions which can be mistaken for eczema. This matters if the wrong treatment is then given. Some of the diseases that can be misdiagnosed as eczema (with the more common ones listed first) are shown in *Box 2.1*.

2.9 What are the complications of eczema?

Bacterial infection

Intact skin is usually very good at keeping out infection but if eczema is present bacterial infection can occur. This is especially common in atopic eczema, where rough or broken skin leads to a much higher level of colonization by staphylococci. The infected areas will look different, with the appearance of pustules (these have green or yellow contents), large blisters with clear or milky contents (impetigo), tender redness and, perhaps, general upset with a raised temperature if the bacteria get in beyond the

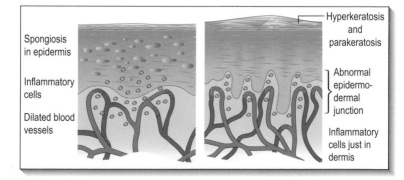

Spongiosis in epidermis

Inflammatory cells

Dilated blood vessels

Hyperkeratosis and parakeratosis

Abnormal epidermo-dermal junction

Inflammatory cells just in dermis

Fig. 2.2 Acute versus chronic eczema.

BOX 2.1 Diseases that can be diagnosed as eczema

Scabies	Itchy persons in close contact, male genitals affected, burrows
Psoriasis	Well-defined borders to patches, silvery scales
Fungal infection	On hands and feet, often one side only; on body, patches usually ring shaped; in scalp, hair is lost.
Candidal infection	Usually in moist body folds, with pustules beyond the red edge
Lichen planus	Shiny purplish flat-topped papules
Drug reaction	Onset soon after beginning a new medicine; does not look typical for eczema
Bullous pemphigoid	Large blisters
Dermatitis herpetiformis	Clusters of small very itchy vesicles, most commonly on knees, elbows and buttocks.

---

skin. If the infection is due to staphylococcus, the toxin produced can lead to a general flare-up of the patient's eczema by acting as a 'superantigen'. This triggers a vicious cycle from triggering of the immune system to release inflammatory cytokines and other chemicals which produce more inflammation, a clinical flare of the eczema and greater opportunities for infection (*Fig. 2.3*).

Herpes simplex infection
In the atopic person, the cold sore virus herpes simplex can produce a much more widespread outbreak of grouped vesicles which break down to

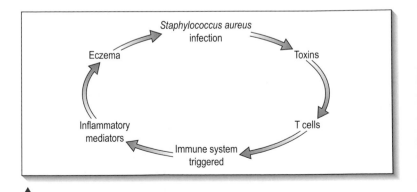

Fig. 2.3 Cycle of infection and inflammation leading to general flare-up of eczema.

produce little erosions. In a baby this can be a serious infection – eczema herpeticum – needing systemic antiviral treatment. Affected patients should be discussed immediately with a dermatologist as they may need admission and intravenous treatment to start with.

Allergic reaction to treatment
If eczema gets worse rather than better with a treatment, this could be because allergy has developed to one or more of the ingredients in the cream or ointment. This is especially likely to occur with eczema on the lower legs due to a disorder of the veins (*see Q 2.5*). The allergy can be due to active materials such as hydrocortisone, antiseptics or antibiotics, and also to chemicals in the base such as the preservative.

Erythroderma (exfoliative dermatitis)
With some kinds of eczema the skin can become red all over, and it is often scaly as well. This situation is called erythroderma if the redness predominates, or exfoliative dermatitis if there is prominent scaling. Other skin diseases (e.g. psoriasis, drug reaction) can become generalized and produce a very similar end result. When the entire skin is affected, various problems can occur: normal temperature regulation can be lost, excessive fluid is lost through the skin, there is strain on the heart – and heart failure can occur. This is another situation in which hospital admission is necessary.

2.10 Are there any useful investigations in the diagnosis of eczema?

This will depend on how certain you are of the diagnosis of eczema, what type of eczema you may have diagnosed and whether there are any suspected complications. For example, if there is a possibility that the rash is not eczema but a fungal infection, then scrapings should be taken and sent to a mycology laboratory (*see Fig. 7.1*). If the eczema might be a result of contact allergy, then referral for patch testing at a dermatology department should be considered. This specialized procedure entails application of selected substances to the skin of the back, and observation for a reaction which mimics the eczema. Bacterial and viral swabs should also be taken if infection is a possibility.

2.11 What about tests for food allergy?

Despite being one of the commonest things patients ask about, food allergy is rarely the cause of eczema. It may only be a problem in some infants with an early onset of atopic eczema and much less so for adults. It can be very difficult to diagnose and the best 'test' is to work with a dietitian who can advise on avoidance followed by challenge.

Many patients seem convinced that eggs or milk do cause them problems and report benefit from avoiding those foods. One possible explanation may be that the lining of the gut can become inflamed when eczema is severe and larger proteins than normal can get through. These larger proteins may trigger an immune response and cause further exacerbation, but once the eczema has settled the gut returns to normal and the larger proteins are kept out.

As with many allergies, diagnosis does need the demonstration of benefit from withdrawing the suspected food, relapse when it is reinstated in the diet and remission when it is again withdrawn.

2.12 Can anything be done to prevent eczema developing?

This question can be taken in several ways. In the sense of primary prevention, the issue is whether some action can be taken to prevent eczema occurring at all in someone who is predicted to develop it. This question has been looked at in respect of atopic families. Some of the interventions tried have included the expectant mother avoiding certain foods during pregnancy, the role of breast feeding, the baby avoiding certain foods, measures to reduce exposure to house dust mite, and avoidance of exposure to pets. The results are not clear cut, partly because such studies are difficult to do, and those taking part have to be studied for many years to find out whether eczema is delayed or truly prevented. So far, there is no good evidence that eczema can be prevented by the expectant mother modifying her diet. Although breast feeding is good for several reasons, it may not prevent eczema. For the very motivated breast feeding mother, her avoidance of milk, dairy products, eggs, fish, peanuts and soya may reduce the severity of eczema in the baby later. There is some evidence that a package of measures including avoidance of milk, with a hydrolysed formula as substitute, and a house dust mite reduction programme during the first few years of life, can reduce the likelihood of eczema. Potential problems with dietary manipulation include the need for supervision by a dietitian and the unpalatability of the hydrolysed formula milk substitutes. In such circumstances it may be worth trying a soya product or milk from a different mammal (e.g. goat or sheep).

For the atopic person, there are other preventive measures that may help. If the family does not have furry pets, it may be sensible not to acquire any, and avoidance of potential irritants such as bubble bath and wool next to the skin is well worthwhile.

Recently there have been reports that feeding infants at risk with probiotics – harmless bacteria such as lactobacilli – can reduce the likelihood of eczema developing. There may also be some benefits from expectant mothers taking them in the later stages of pregnancy and when breast feeding. Further studies and a longer period of observation are needed to know if this measure can be widely recommended, but it is probably worth suggesting to prospective parents with a strong family history of atopic eczema.

For anyone with eczema where specific triggers have been identified, avoidance of these may prevent relapse or worsening.

2.13 What are the principles of management?

The essentials are:

- Make a diagnosis, or range of possible diagnoses, which can be evaluated by some tests if necessary.
- Establish what anxieties and questions the patient or family has and the degree of impact on quality of life (loss of sleep, school, work, etc.).
- Explore what makes the eczema worse. These questions can sometimes lead to useful tests, and often point to measures that will help (e.g. protect the skin with a pure grease when in the swimming pool).
- Emollients. For dryness, use emollients. These can be in the form of creams, ointments and oils dispersed in the bath. Relieving dryness may also help itch. The best emollient is the one that feels best – this may require trying a few. Emollients based on grease alone (e.g. soft white paraffin) and emulsifying ointment are often very well tolerated, i.e. do not sting or irritate, but are less cosmetically attractive.
- A soap substitute. For use in the bath or shower there are dispersible oils which not only help to make skin less dry but also cleanse. Aqueous cream, emulsifying ointment and some other emollients can also be used as soap substitutes.
- Treat infection if it occurs. This is a common reason for eczema getting worse, and a suitable antibiotic should clear it up.
- A topical steroid. Most eczema will improve with a suitable topical steroid. This should be sufficiently potent to produce real benefit but should not used for longer than necessary. The issue of safety is dealt with in *Question 2.14*.

2.14 Can topical steroids be used safely?

Before answering this it is useful to summarize some of the undesirable effects that can occur with use of topical steroids. These are in the skin itself: thinning, easy bruising, skin fragility, stretch marks, easily visible dilated blood vessels and the masking of infection. If a steroid is applied over a large proportion of the body surface, enough can be absorbed to suppress the body's production of cortisol; in children, growth retardation can occur.

Several factors will determine the likelihood of side effects occurring:

■ *The potency of the steroid*: There is a large difference in both effectiveness and side effects between the weakest and most potent – perhaps a 20-fold difference. The weakest are unlikely to produce side effects if used correctly.

■ *The body site*: On some parts of the body the steroid penetrates much more readily and greater caution is needed. Vulnerable areas include the face, neck, major skin creases (armpits and groins) and genital areas.

■ *Occlusive covering*: If there is a non-breathable layer over the steroid-treated skin, the penetration of the steroid will be much greater. Examples include plastic-backed nappies (diapers).

■ *Frequency of application*: The more applications per day, the greater the risk of side effects. In fact, most skin diseases that are treated with steroids will respond satisfactorily to just one application daily.

■ *The duration of treatment*: All the steroid side effects take time to develop – usually longer than the time needed for benefit. When side effects do occur, it is often because the steroid has been continued for too long at the same frequency without any tailing off as the eczema improves. It is generally best to use the steroid for as short a time as possible on a regular continuing basis, then having as long as possible without it – perhaps using the emollient (bland greasy cream or ointment) more often.

The answer to the question posed will therefore depend on what parts of the skin are being treated, which steroid is being used and whether the condition is likely to need treatment long term. It is generally best to use a steroid which is potent enough to work, but not for long enough to produce harmful effects. Because these occur quite quickly on the face, no more than a moderately potent one should be prescribed. The same applies to sites where the skin will be occluded (e.g. the napkin area). A potent steroid can be safe if it is not used continuously for long enough to produce side effects – perhaps 2–3 weeks. A weaker steroid (or if possible an emollient) may then be used if necessary to maintain improvement.

The topical steroids vary greatly in potency, perhaps by a factor of 20-fold between the weakest and the strongest. All those available can be placed in one of four categories (*Box 2.2*). Skin side effects are mainly associated with the potent and very potent steroids.

2.15 What is tachyphylaxis?

This is a phenomenon where repeated use of a treatment, in this case topical steroids, can lead to loss of effect. It is a reason not to continue using a particular potency of preparation longer than is absolutely necessary. For some patients who do need topical steroids for a prolonged period, it can be made less likely if they use emollients alone on 1 or 2 days a week.

BOX 2.2 Topical corticosteroid potencies	
Potency	Examples
Mild	Hydrocortisone acetate 1%
Moderately potent	Aclometasone dipropionate 0.05%
	Clobetasone butyrate 0.05%
	Dexamethasone 0.05%
Potent	Betamethasone dipropionate 0.05%
	Betamethasone valerate 0.1%
	Fluocinonide 0.05%
	Fluticasone propionate 0.05%
	Hydrocortisone 17-butyrate 0.1%
	Mometasone furoate 0.1%
Very potent	Clobetasol propionate 0.05%
	Halcinonide 0.1%

2.16 Are there any specific treatments for some of the different types of eczema?

If there is a cause – such as exposure to an irritant or allergen – avoidance of it is an essential part of the treatment. Similarly, if eczema on the lower leg is due to raised pressure in the leg veins (*see Fig. 10.1*), then support hosiery or surgery (if feasible) can cure the eczema.

If the eczema is seborrhoeic in type, then treatment will be more effective if it includes an ingredient which reduces or eliminates the contributory surface yeasts.

When eczema is aggravated by bacterial infection, the addition of a suitable antibiotic will not only clear up the infection but may also help the eczema to settle. Systemic antibiotics may be better than topical ones as sensitization can be a problem. Once the infection has cleared, the antibiotic should be stopped. There are some topical preparations containing an antibiotic and a steroid but they should only be used in the short term to avoid the added problem of resistance.

2.17 What about the newer immunomodulatory drugs?

For the last 50 years the most effective topical treatments we have had for eczema have been the topical steroids, which work by their effects on the immune system in the skin. Recently two new products have become available which are effective for eczema, and work by suppressing the skin immune system; however, they are not corticosteroids, being referred to as calcineurin inhibitors. These are Protopic 0.1 and 0.03% ointments which contain tacrolimus and Elidel cream whose active ingredient is pimecrolimus; these work in a similar way to each other but are unlike topical steroids and do not thin the skin. They are most likely to be useful in situations where topical steroids can be problematic – for example on the face and body folds when the weakest steroids are not effective, and where potent topical steroids do not seem to be working, perhaps because of tachyphylaxis. In the future, these products may be used in conjunction with steroids to produce specific management plans for individual patients.

2.18 When can bandages be useful?

Bandaging for eczema provides some protection from scratching and rubbing and, if the process produces occlusion, there will be increased hydration. If a topical steroid is used with the bandaging, its potency will be enhanced. Currently, wet bandaging for eczema means either the use of a paste-impregnated cotton open-weave bandage underneath a lightweight elasticated cotton tubular layer or a cream (or ointment) on the skin followed by wet and dry layers of the elasticated cotton tubing (wet wrapping). The cotton open-weave bandage can be impregnated with a bland preparation such as zinc paste, or have an active ingredient like ichthammol or coal tar.

Bandaging can be useful when the techniques for doing it are well understood and there is supervision from someone like a dermatological specialist nurse. There are, however, potential hazards: hypothermia, enhanced infection risk and increased absorption of any steroid used. The generous use of a very weak steroid cream beneath the wet layer in a wet wrap can be a useful short term part of the management of acute eczema. This can usefully be followed by emollient alone under the two layers. Wet wrapping is probably of most use for children whose sleep (and that of their parents) is disrupted by scratching. A few nights' sleep can break a cycle of itching and scratching and improve the quality of life for the whole family.

Paste bandaging is usually used for more subacute or chronic eczema. Particularly for the latter, a tar (ichthammol or coal tar) can be effective with or without a weak steroid.

2.19 Are antihistamines useful in eczema?

Sedative antihistamines (e.g. hydroxyzine, alimemazine and promethazine) at night are a safe way of prescribing a hypnotic. Some infants become paradoxically hyperactive and tachyphylaxis may occur so it is best to use these drugs in short courses. Although there is no good evidence that the itch in eczema is due to histamine, and non-sedative H1 antagonists are not generally of value, some patients do benefit. This may be because some of the inflammatory change in the skin is a type 1 reaction against common environmental allergens such as the house dust mite. There is no evidence that H2 antihistamines are of any use in eczema.

2.20 What dose and duration of treatment are needed when treating infection with antibiotics?

To eradicate pathogenic staphylococci (and streptococci when present) from the skin can require a higher dose and a longer treatment time than is needed for some internal infections. An example would be the dose of flucloxacillin in adults of 500 mg q.d.s. for 10–14 days. It is, of course, necessary to treat the eczema at the same time. If there is little or no response, take a swab to check the sensitivities of the staphylococcus.

2.21 When should patients be referred to hospital?

Occasionally referral to hospital is needed as a matter of urgency – for example, severe bacterial infection not responding to treatment, eczema herpeticum in an infant and eczema that is involving almost all the skin (erythroderma) so as to cause systemic upset.

Otherwise, hospital referral is likely to be for confirmation of diagnosis when this is not straightforward, for investigations (e.g. patch testing) when contact allergy is a possibility, or for consideration of treatments that are hospital based or require supervision by a dermatologist. If dietary modification is to be tried, it may be necessary to have advice from a hospital-based dietitian (*see Q 2.11*). The atopic individual may also need help from hospital services for problems relating to asthma and allergies (e.g. gastrointestinal, ocular, rhinitis, etc.).

2.22 Are there any good practice guidelines about referring patients?

The National Institute for Clinical Excellence (NICE), as well as investigating the value of various treatments, has produced referral guidelines (*see Appendix*). One of these is for the management of children with atopic eczema. In this document it is accepted that 'most children with atopic eczema can be managed in primary care' but then lists reasons for referral to a specialist service as:

- Severe infection with herpes simplex (eczema herpeticum) is suspected
- The disease is severe and has not responded to appropriate therapy in primary care
- The rash becomes infected with bacteria and treatment with an oral antibiotic plus a topical corticosteroid has failed
- Treatment requires the use of excessive amounts of potent topical corticosteroids
- Management in primary care has not controlled the rash satisfactorily. Ultimately, failure to improve is probably best based on a subjective assessment by the child or parent

- The patient or family might benefit from additional advice on application of treatments (bandaging techniques)
- Contact dermatitis is suspected and confirmation requires patch testing
- Dietary factors are suspected and dietary control a possibility
- The diagnosis is, or has become, uncertain.

It is worth noting that not all of these require a consultant dermatologist. For example, a specialist dermatology nurse would be appropriate for advice on bandaging techniques.

2.23 What different treatments are used in hospital?

If admission is needed because of infection, the appropriate antibiotic or antiviral drug may well be given intravenously to begin with. If the eczema is very widespread, patients often benefit by being relieved of the chore of applying treatments – this will be done by nurses with knowledge of the skin and its diseases. If the eczema is acute and weeping, soaks or compresses followed by creams – sometimes in conjunction with moist bandaging – will be used until the eczema settles down. For eczema that is dry, greasier creams or ointments will be used to moisturize the skin. This type of treatment approach can often be carried out in a day centre, avoiding the need for admission and allowing patients to live as normal a life as possible.

Sometimes eczema is too severe for topical therapy to bring it under control. The hospital dermatology department may then offer phototherapy or systemic treatment. Phototherapy consists of exposure to ultraviolet (UV) radiation. Currently most dermatologists use a form called narrowband UVB; longer wavelength UVA in conjunction with a photosensitizing medicine called psoralen (the combination is called PUVA) is also used (*see Q 4.19*). Internal treatments to suppress eczema include oral corticosteroids (rarely used other than for short periods) and immunosuppressant medicine. These can be very effective, but supervision is needed for various unwanted effects that can occur. This supervision will entail regular blood tests. The most commonly used immunosuppressants are ciclosporin and azathioprine.

2.24 Are there any new treatments being developed?

Current topical treatments are far from ideal; they are often time consuming, can be messy, and may not control the eczema sufficiently. There will be anxieties about some of them – for example, the stronger steroids. The systemic treatments that are effective all have some risk. There is much need for something better.

From what we know of the mechanisms that underlie eczema, there are likely to be new developments. In atopic eczema there is a disorder of cyclic nucleotide metabolism, and it has been predicted that phosphodiesterase inhibitors may be effective – time and well-conducted clinical trials will tell. In a recent controlled trial it was found that feeding harmless lactobacilli can help atopic eczema (*see Q 2.12*); however, more experience is needed before we can comment on the usefulness of this approach.

 PATIENT QUESTIONS

2.25 What is the best moisturizer for me to use?

The best moisturizer is the one you *will* use! Greasy preparations may be the best but are no use to you if you cannot get along with them. There is no easy answer to your question, you just have to try a range of different products and make your mind up. Your doctor might have some sample products or you could pick some up at one of the skin information days run by the Skin Care Campaign (*see Appendix*). It may well be that you will end up with several different moisturizers for use on different parts of your body and at different times of the day. For example, if you use a keyboard you will not want a very greasy product on your hands during the day but might be able to use a greasier one at night. One thing to remember is that the lighter and less greasy a product is, the more frequently you will need to apply it.

2.26 How should I apply a moisturizer?

You should smooth it onto the skin going with the direction of hair growth, where you have hair. Avoid rubbing it in too vigorously as this often irritates the skin and makes it more itchy. If you can allow it time to soak in, do this as it will last longer.

2.27 Some moisturizers seem to sting or irritate my skin – does this mean I am allergic to them?

Not necessarily. When your skin is inflamed, almost anything will feel irritating when you first put it on. Apply it gently and do not rub in and any initial stinging should settle. It is certainly possible to be allergic to some of the components – especially the preservatives – so discuss any persisting problems with your doctor. Greasy products tend to be less likely to sting than creamy ones.

2.28 Why won't my doctor allow me to use a strong steroid on my face? It works really well.

The skin on your face, in common with skin in flexures, is thinner and much more likely to suffer side effects from steroids. These include permanent problems like thinning and stretch marks and also problems like acne that would need different treatments. On the face, you should also be particularly careful around the eyes as steroids applied close to them can be absorbed and lead to increased pressure in the eyes (glaucoma) and cataracts.

2.29 What does patch testing involve?

Patch testing involves three trips to the hospital department in 1 week. Various products, including well-known sensitizers and anything you suspect you might be allergic to, will be applied to your back in little discs secured with tape. You might have 20–30 discs which are left in place for 2 days and then removed. Any reaction is checked immediately and in a further 2 days. The doctor or nurse will then give you a list of anything that you might be allergic to along with guidance about what products or substances you should avoid.

2.30 My eczema always gets better when I am on holiday, why is this?

This could be from a combination of factors. Firstly, you might simply be more relaxed and less stressed on holiday. Secondly the environment might be different – more sun, less house dust mite, different diet, etc. Thirdly, you could be avoiding something at work that might be causing your eczema – this should lead you to suspect an allergic reaction.

2.31 Can I use any make-up or perfume products without making my eczema worse?

You should be able to find some products you can use. Some companies make a 'hypoallergenic' range which means that you might be less likely to develop a reaction. A good test to do with any new product is to apply it to some of your skin that doesn't have any eczema and that wouldn't be too much of a problem if a reaction was caused. This could be the inside of your arm. Use a small amount of the new product there for a few days and, if it doesn't react, it should be OK. Patient groups such as the National Eczema Society (*see Appendix*) could give you further advice about this.

2.32 I have been told I am allergic to nickel – is it just cheap jewellery I need to avoid?

No, unfortunately nickel is present in many common items made of, or containing, metal:

- Clothes fastenings such as jeans studs, hooks and zips
- Other personal objects – cigarette lighters, wristwatches, key rings, keys, parts of spectacle frames and pens
- Household items such as drawer and cupboard handles, kitchen utensils and toasters, etc.
- Silver coins.

The list could almost be endless so only a few examples are given above. There is also the added problem of the nickel content of some foods from natural sources or in the way they are prepared. This can be a problem if you have a severe reaction to nickel. Avoid canned foods and use aluminium or stainless steel utensils when cooking. A dietitian could give you a list of foods to avoid which would include asparagus, oysters, herrings (other fish are OK), mushrooms, onions, tomatoes and rhubarb.

Acne

3

3.1   What is acne?

Acne is a disease of the pilosebaceous apparatus comprising inflammatory and non-inflammatory lesions, the latter being known as comedones. Ordinary acne is more properly known as acne vulgaris. There are other types of acne – for example, those due to exposure to oil, certain hydrocarbons, etc. Acne is associated with an increased sebum excretion rate.

The comedones (blackheads and whiteheads) are a result of abnormal formation and a failure of shedding of the horny layer (stratum corneum) within the opening of the pilosebaceous duct, and retention of sebum and squames in a cyst-like swelling just beneath the surface of the skin. Inflammation, largely due to the presence of the commensal bacterium *Propionibacterium acnes* which thrives in the lipid-rich comedo, results in papules, pustules, nodules and large collections of pus, sometimes (wrongly) called cysts. When the inflammation settles there may be various types of scarring and true epidermal cysts (*Fig. 3.1*).

Acne occurs on body sites where there are numerous pilosebaceous units – notably the face, back, chest and shoulders.

3.2   How long does acne last?

This is such an important question for the individual enduring acne, but one that cannot be answered for that individual. Most acne lasts at least a few years.

3.3   Is acne always a disease of teenagers?

No. Although it usually starts between the ages of 12 and 14 years and peaks around 16–17 years for girls and 17–19 years for boys, acne does persist into

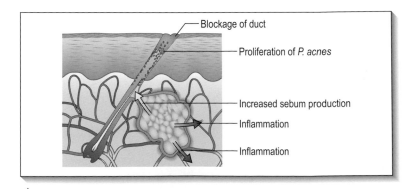

Blockage of duct

Proliferation of *P. acnes*

Increased sebum production

Inflammation

Inflammation

▲

Fig. 3.1 The pilosebaceous unit in acne.

the 20s and beyond. Some people only start to develop it after their teenage years and tend to have a less responsive type. Some 15% of women in their 40s are still troubled by acne.

There is also an infantile form which is much rarer. It presents soon after birth and may be the result of maternal androgens crossing the placenta and stimulating sebaceous glands. It is more common in boys, can last up to 3 years and may indicate that those affected will develop severe acne in adolescence.

3.4 What is the difference between acne and rosacea?

Rosacea has nothing to do with acne: it is not centred on pilosebaceous units, and is not associated with increased sebum production or with *P. acnes*. It is thus misleading to refer to the condition by the old name of 'acne rosacea'. In rosacea there are papules and sterile pustules on a background of erythema and telangiectasia. There is often flushing, which can precede other features of the disorder. There are no comedones. Rosacea usually occurs on the convex areas of the forehead, cheeks, nose and chin. In the long term, persistent swelling of the skin may occur. Eye symptoms are common, and sometimes potentially serious keratitis can occur. It does, however, respond to antibiotics – topical metronidazole or oral tetracyclines.

3.5 Is perioral dermatitis a form of acne?

No, perioral dermatitis is an inflammatory condition distinct from acne and rosacea. It occurs mainly in young women. The eruption consists of tiny papules and pustules, usually on a red background, typically arranged around the mouth. Sometimes lesions occur on the eyelids and glabella. There are no comedones, no increased sebum production and *P. acnes* is not involved. Many but not all cases are related to the use of topical steroids on the face. Once again, there is similarity in the type of treatment – usually 6 weeks to 3 months of oral tetracyclines.

3.6 What features would suggest gram-negative folliculitis?

Worsening of acne in a patient on long-term antibiotics, particularly when there is a sudden outbreak of pustules, is a characteristic presentation. Lesions may also be more deep seated and nodular. A variety of Gram-negative bacilli can produce this condition. If suspected, send a swab from pustule contents. The best treatment is usually oral isotretinoin. If this is not an option, amoxicillin is usually effective.

3.7 What is acne fulminans?

This term is used to describe a systemic illness due to an excessive immunological response to the acne bacillus, *P. acnes*. Typically there is rapid onset of widespread severe inflammatory acne together with fever, malaise, weight loss, anorexia and multiple bone and joint pains. Patients have a marked leucocytosis and lytic bone lesions. Occasionally this rare condition is triggered by Epstein–Barr virus and it has also been associated with testosterone treatment. The acne is usually treated with oral isotretinoin and the systemic disease with prednisolone.

3.8 Does acne develop because the skin is too greasy?

Although acne occurs in individuals who have a high rate of sebum excretion, the grease lying on the surface of the skin does not cause the acne. Paradoxically, the individual pilosebaceous units in which comedones and then other manifestations of acne occur will eventually have no output of sebum – because they have become blocked. The main driving force for sebum production and excretion is the presence of androgenic hormones, levels of which are not necessarily raised. The pilosebaceous unit in acne is much more sensitive to normal circulating levels of androgens than in normal skin and produces more sebum. The ducts become blocked because of overgrowth of epithelium and clumping of the shed keratinocytes. This blockage and the excess amount of sebum creates an excellent environment for the growth of *P. acnes* bacteria resulting in inflammation and collection of pus.

3.9 Does diet affect acne?

Medical science and the patient's belief frequently part company over this question. Although it was widely taught in the 1950s that acne was due to food, especially certain fats and chocolate, and many sufferers have similar beliefs today, there is no good evidence that intake of carbohydrate, lipids or any other dietary factors is important in general.

3.10 What are the different lesions in acne?

Microcomedones represent the initial lesion when the blockage occurs and they can progress into larger comedones or rupture at an early stage, leading to inflammatory lesions. Comedones can be either closed (whiteheads) or open (blackheads). The black appearance of open comedones is not to do with dirt – it is due to the skin pigment melanin in the duct. Inflamed lesions are either papules or pustules. Papules tend to occur when a blocked duct ruptures and leaks sebum into the surrounding tissue. When this happens at the microcomedonal stage, papules appear without the usual crop of visible comedones. Pustules arise from infection within the duct.

Nodules and 'cysts' tend to be deeper lesions that affect the dermis, and so result in scarring. Nodules are solid and inflammatory and occur in the same way as papules when a larger comedone ruptures. What are referred to as 'cysts' are really the clustering of two or three nodules which break down to form bags of pus.

3.11 Can treatment be matched to the pattern and type of acne?

To some extent, yes. The choice made depends on the severity of the acne (*Table 3.1*), its location, rate of progress and extent, and treatments used so far (*Table 3.2*). It also takes account of the psychological impact of the acne on the patient.

3.12 How do you decide what treatments to use?

Several criteria contribute to the decision as to which treatment(s) to use:

■ With the exception of isotretinoin, appropriate combinations of acne treatments can often be superior to single agents.
■ All oral acne treatments are slow to work so patients need to be encouraged to stick with them, generally for several months, before

TABLE 3.1 Severity of acne

	Mild	Moderate	Severe
Comedones	+ to ++	+ to +++	+ to +++
Papules	0 to ++	0 to +++	+ to +++
Pustules	0 to ++	0 to +++	+ to +++
Nodules	0	0	+ to +++
Cysts	0	0	+ to +++
Scars	0	0	+ to +++
Treatments	Topical ? + oral antibiotic	Topical agent + oral antibiotic, and/or in females co-cyprindiol	Isotretinoin

TABLE 3.2 Treatment of acne

Lesions	Topical treatment	Oral treatment
Comedones	Topical retinoid	Isotretinoin
Papules	Benzoyl peroxide, adapalene, nicotinamide	Tetracyclines
Pustules	Azelaic acid, topical antibiotics	Erythromycin, trimethoprim, co-cyprindiol, isotretinoin
Nodules	Short-term superpotent topical steroid, intralesional corticosteroid	Isotretinoin
'Cysts'	None	Isotretinoin
Scars	Haelan tape for hypertrophic scars and keloids	Cosmetic camouflage Resurfacing techniques

much improvement is likely and it is often open ended as to how long the treatment will be needed.

- There are relatively few good comparative studies to help narrow the choice among the topical agents. The topical antibiotics are associated with the development of resistant *P. acnes* (*see* Q 3.13). It is not sensible to use the combination of a topical and an oral antibiotic.

- Topical agents with different properties can be used together – for example, a retinoid at night for its action against comedones and benzoyl peroxide in the morning for its anti-inflammatory and antibacterial effect (*Fig. 3.2*).

- Severely inflammatory destructive acne should be considered sooner rather than later for treatment with oral isotretinoin.

Although we can be objective about the severity of acne, the patient's own view is most important and can swing the balance as to which treatments should be used. If there is disproportionate psychological upset and even dysmorphophobia, it may be appropriate to consider isotretinoin much sooner than otherwise.

3.13 Is there a problem with drug resistance?

The *P. acnes* bacteria do become resistant to antibiotics and this can lead to a lack of response. As acne is not primarily caused by infection this is often not as much of a problem as it could be. Other treatments can kill the bacteria, especially benzoyl peroxide, and one way to combat resistance is to use this along with oral antibiotics. Even if the patient does not want to use it all the time, a week's course every 4 weeks will mop up resistant bacteria and improve the efficacy of the antibiotic. Some topical antibiotic preparations contain zinc as this is also thought to help counter resistance.

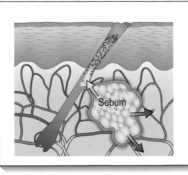

Reduce hyperkeratinization:
retinoids

Antibacterial effect:
benzoyl peroxide, topical antibiotics, oral antibiotics

Decrease sebum production:
retinoids, antiandrogens

Reduce inflammation:
antibiotics, intralesional corticosteroids

Sebum

▲

Fig. 3.2 The pilosebaceous unit showing the sites of action of acne drugs.

3.14 How long should treatment last?

The easiest answer is for oral isotretinoin, which for most patients will take for 4–6 months and the patient may not need acne treatment thereafter. For topical treatments the course is open ended and if acne recurs on discontinuing, more treatment is needed. Oral antibiotics are not now given for such long courses as they used to be, so patients should be reassessed after a maximum of 6 months.

There are concerns with long-term continuous use of co-cyprindiol (Dianette) which is no longer recommended for use just as a contraceptive as it may carry a higher risk of cerebrovascular accident than lower dose 'standard' oral contraceptives. The current recommendation is to discontinue co-cyprindiol 3–4 months after acne is cleared, and switch to an alternative contraceptive if that effect was also desired – although a further course can be given again if necessary.

If minocycline is given long term, it is recommended that liver tests and antinuclear antibodies (because of possible hepatotoxicity and drug-induced lupus erythematosus) are checked 3 monthly and the skin checked for blue–grey pigmentation.

3.15 When should be patients be referred to hospital?

The National Institute for Clinical Excellence (NICE, *see Appendix*) has produced a guideline for referral of acne patients to a specialist service. This acknowledges that most patients with acne can be managed in primary care but that they should be referred if they:

■ have a severe variant of acne such as gram-negative folliculitis (*see Q 3.6*) or acne fulminans (*see Q 3.7*)
■ have severe or nodulocystic acne and could benefit from oral isotretinoin
■ have severe social or psychological problems, including a morbid fear of deformity (dysmorphophobia)
■ are at risk of, or are developing, scarring despite primary care therapies
■ have moderate acne that has failed to respond to treatment which has included two courses of oral antibiotics, each lasting 3 months; failure is probably best based upon a subjective assessment by the patient
■ are suspected of having an underlying endocrinological cause for the acne (e.g. polycystic ovary syndrome) that needs assessment
■ have, or develop, features that make the diagnosis uncertain.

It is interesting that NICE emphasize a subjective view of failure so it is important to listen to the patient's view on success and not just to judge it on clinical grounds.

3.16 What different treatments are used in hospital?

Oral isotretinoin is only licensed in the UK for prescription by consultant dermatologists although this is not the case in some other parts of the world. Consultants also have much more experience of using higher doses of antibiotics and some of the less commonly used ones such as trimethoprim.

Other treatments that may be available in secondary care include steroid injection of scars and isolated nodulocystic lesions, electrocautery of large comedones, cosmetic camouflage advice, resurfacing lasers, chemical peels, dermabrasion and injection of fillers for depressed scars (*see Qs 3.20 and 3.21*).

3.17 Does oral isotretinoin cause depression?

There are anecdotal reports and small published series of patients becoming depressed while on or shortly after taking oral isotretinoin. The data sheet warns of this, and the possibility of suicide. There have been 37 cases of suicide out of 5 million people who have taken isotretinoin in the USA, but this is no greater than the expected suicide rate in a matched population. When the occurrence of depression in acne patients treated with isotretinoin has been compared with those treated with oral antibiotics there has been no difference. If the problem does exist, it is not clear how great it is and whether a pre-existing depressive or other psychiatric illness is a risk factor. With all this uncertainty it seems sensible to ask about mood change before and during isotretinoin treatment. In the UK the Acne Support Group (*see Appendix*) suggests that vulnerable patients living on their own with no close support from family and friends should be monitored closely if they are prescribed isotretinoin.

3.18 What are the side effects of isotretinoin?

Isotretinoin is teratogenic. It is therefore of the greatest importance that females of child-bearing potential taking isotretinoin are not pregnant at the onset of treatment and do not become pregnant until at least 4 weeks after the course is completed. Most patients taking isotretinoin will have one or more of the commoner side effects but it is generally possible to ameliorate these, either with some symptomatic remedies or if necessary by modifying the dose. There is no problem with men taking the drug whilst trying to get their partners pregnant.

Other side effects of isotretinoin are listed in *Box 3.1*. It is very important that patients are fully counselled about the possible side effects and know

BOX 3.1 Side effects of isotretinoin

Side effects	Treatment
Cheilitis	Lubricant, e.g. soft or hard paraffin – if severe, add a mild steroid ointment
Nasal dryness	Soft paraffin
Dry skin	Emollient – if necessary add a mild topical steroid for itch
Blepharoconjunctivitis	Ocular lubricant – mild steroid/antibiotic combination if necessary
Dermatitis/eczema	Emollient and mild/moderate topical steroid
Photosensitivity	Sunscreen and sun protection measures
Arthalgia and myalgia	Paracetamol and/or non-steroidal anti-inflammatory drug
Headache	Paracetamol – if severe, consider benign intracranial hypertension and stop treatment

how to cope with them. Although the drug is prescribed in hospital, GPs must also be familiar with the potential problems and solutions. Arthralgia and myalgia are usually only a problem for very active patients training for or participating in sport on a regular basis.

One problem that does occur is an apparent worsening of the acne in the first few weeks. This can be very distressing for patients as they will have built up their hopes for great benefits from the treatment, only to find their acne is, at best, no better for the first month or two of treatment whilst the side effects are apparent almost immediately. Most of the benefit seems to be in the second half of the course (*Fig. 3.3*).

3.19 What if a patient relapses after isotretinoin?

There is about a 60% chance of acne being cured or only trivial after an adequate course of oral isotretinoin. Some research papers use the measure of need for any further oral medication as a sign of relapse so patients do often need some topical treatments to 'finish off' their acne. As the retinoid is especially good at treating comedones, topical treatments such as benzoyl peroxide and antibiotics are usually the first ones to try.

Of those who do relapse, many will have acne of a lower level of severity which will respond better to other treatments than it did before the isotretinoin. Probably about 20% will have at least one further course of oral isotretinoin. A few patients will need several courses to achieve remission.

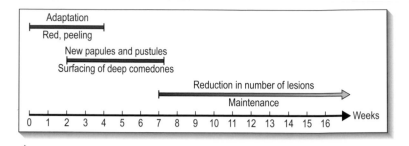

Fig. 3.3 Expected skin changes during a course of isotretinoin. (Reproduced from Habif T P 2004 Clinical dermatology: a colour guide to diagnosis and treatment, 4th edn. Mosby, Edinburgh, with kind permission from Elsevier.)

3.20 Are there any good treatments for scarring?

There are many types of scar after inflammatory acne has settled. Excessive collagen deposition produces the hypertrophic scar (these eventually flatten) and the keloid (this does not resolve, and can continue enlarging over time). Loss of tissue can produce the so-called ice-pick scar, irregularities of contour of the skin, flat white scars, and focal white perifollicular lesions. Scars can, and often do, improve with the passage of time.

If it is clear that a hypertrophic scar or keloid is not improving, a potent topical steroid carefully applied for a few weeks may help, and if not, an intralesional steroid injection is often of value. Vascular keloids can be helped by the pulsed-dye laser (*see Q 3.21*).

A few prominent deep ice-pick scars can often be improved by excision. Flat or nearly flat scars can sometimes be improved by resurfacing lasers (e.g. ultrapulsed carbon dioxide, neodymium:YAG and erbium:YAG). In the right hands, the older techniques of chemical peeling and dermabrasion may be successful but can produce scarring in their own right – as well as unsightly pigmentary problems. Undulating indentations can be filled with collagen and some newer materials, but repeated injections are needed and some of the agents used provoke unwanted reactions.

Patients should be advised to be cautious before proceeding with any treatments for scarring, especially if exaggerated claims of success are being made. Professional bodies such as the British Association of Dermatologists (*see Appendix*) or the British Association of Plastic Surgeons can help with the choice of a reputable practitioner.

3.21 What about light or laser treatment?

A laser emits a single wavelength of coherent light. Lasers and some other non-coherent light sources are being used in the treatment of acne, mainly in the commercial sector. Photodynamic therapy (in which a porphyrin precursor is applied followed by exposure to light) is also being used. Some of these treatments have been evaluated in controlled trials, but there are few adequate comparisons with other treatments.

Mild/moderate inflammatory acne has been effectively treated with the pulsed-dye laser, the 1450 mm diode laser, blue light, blue plus red light and photodynamic therapy. There are probably different modes of action for these diverse treatments and further studies are needed before they can be routinely recommended. More severe grades of acne have either been excluded from the studies, or clearly shown not to respond.

Laser treatments have been used for some of the scarring that can follow acne; these include the pulsed-dye, ultrapulsed carbon dioxide, neodymium:YAG and erbium:YAG lasers.

 PATIENT QUESTIONS

3.22 What does my GP mean when he says my acne is 'moderate'?

There are several different ways of grading acne; some are very complex and are used for research purposes to evaluate the benefit of a treatment. Very basically, four grades can be used and linked to the type of treatment as shown earlier in this chapter. The grades take into account the types and numbers of the various lesions as well as any scarring which would include pigment changes in darker skin. It may be that different parts of the body merit a different grade (e.g. mild on the face but severe on the back) and the psychological effect will need to be taken into account. If you are very upset by your acne this will put you up a grade compared to just judging it by its appearance.

3.23 Is acne worse in black skin?

The important difference with acne in dark skin is that the inflammatory component is less obvious, but the consequences – post-inflammatory hyperpigmentation producing black patches – are very obvious. Another difference is the higher incidence of keloid scarring. Pomades used to improve the manageability of hair can also produce acne and this should be considered with acne on the forehead and temples.

Because of the pigmentation and keloid scarring, acne in darker skin should be treated aggressively and 'a grade above' its appearance.

3.24 My acne always gets worse just before my periods – what can I do about this?

Acne can fluctuate with periods and you might want to discuss trying a hormonal preparation with your doctor. Dianette contains oestrogen and an agent that blocks androgens and can be useful in this situation. It also acts as a contraceptive so this must be taken into consideration as well.

3.25 I am training to be a chef but find the hot humid conditions in the kitchen make my acne worse. What can I do to prevent this?

It may be difficult to prevent the conditions having some effect on your acne. The following might help:

- Ask if you can work near an open window or other form of ventilation
- Use a cleanser regularly during breaks to help remove any build-up of sweat and grease
- Avoid make-up on your face when at work as this could lead to blocked pores and worsen the problem.

3.26 If retinoids are derived from vitamin A, can I just take vitamin A tablets?

The various retinoid treatments are based on natural or synthetic vitamin A but it is not recommended to take vitamin A itself. Like many 'natural' substances, it can be quite toxic and can damage your liver. This is especially important for children and pregnant women. There have been some trials of low-dose vitamin A but no conclusive benefit has been shown.

Psoriasis

4

4.1 How common is psoriasis?

In Western Europe about 3% of the population have psoriasis. It is less common in those of oriental and West African origin, and rare in the indigenous peoples of the American continent.

4.2 What is the cause of psoriasis?

It is likely that psoriasis can occur only in someone with the appropriate genetic constitution. Psoriasis presenting early in life is, in general, much more likely to have an obvious family history than the later onset form in the 50s or 60s. Psoriasis is not due to a fault in a single gene as several have been identified – perhaps up to 15. Neither is it just caused by genetic abnormalities. This is best illustrated by identical twins as, where one twin has the disease, the incidence in the other twin is only 70% rather than the 100% to be expected on genetic grounds alone.

The strongest association is with HLA-Cw6, although this itself is not the 'psoriasis gene'. Other genes unrelated to HLA, some determining pro-inflammatory cytokines, are also important. It may be that this uncertainty about what genes are involved will be found to help explain the differing patterns of presentation of the disease (*see* Q 4.6).

4.3 If there is a family history, what are the risks for the children?

If one parent has psoriasis, there is approximately a 10% chance of a child developing the condition. This rises to 50% if both parents have it.

4.4 What are the triggers for an outbreak of psoriasis?

Sometimes psoriasis can be triggered by one or more of the following:

- Injury to the skin, e.g. a wound – accidental or surgical
- Infection, especially a sore throat, caused by the bacterium *Streptococcus pyogenes* Group A
- Medicines, e.g. lithium and some antimalarials (chloroquine)
- Alcohol and cigarette smoking
- Emotional upset
- Sunlight can sometimes bring on psoriasis or make it worse
- HIV infection.

4.5 What are the changes that happen within the skin?

For the doctor and the patient new to psoriasis it can be difficult to reconcile that several rather different visible appearances are all part of the same process.

Psoriasis is an inflammatory disorder – there is always redness. This is usually pronounced, and typically well defined, i.e. there is a sharp distinction between the psoriasis and surrounding normal skin. Although psoriasis can begin as a small elevated lesion – a papule – it usually expands to form larger raised plaques. These are covered with silvery scales, unless skin is next to skin (e.g. in body folds when the occlusion prevents the skin from drying out and scaling). There is usually some degree of itching (the term psoriasis means 'a state of being itchy') which can vary from minimal to intolerable.

Histological examination of psoriatic skin shows thickening of the epidermis, mainly due to downward extension of the epidermal ridges. The cells in the horny layer have retained their nuclei – a finding called parakeratosis – so are still living and supplied by dilated and tortuous capillaries which are seen in the dermal papillae. These changes are a result of inflammation, brought about by certain types of white blood cell accumulating in the skin. These include T-lymphocytes, which are mainly in the dermis, and polymorphonuclear neutrophil leucocytes which, when present in sufficient numbers, account for pustules and can be seen histologically as microabscesses. It is likely that the T-lymphocytes infiltrating the upper dermis are the earliest event as they produce various substances (cytokines and other mediators of inflammation) which cause all the other changes. The immature cells of the epidermis are an important source of further molecules which sustain the process (*Fig. 4.1*).

4.6 Are there different patterns of presentation?

It is perplexing that psoriasis can appear so different from person to person, at different body sites, and over time in the same person. The main presentations are as follows.

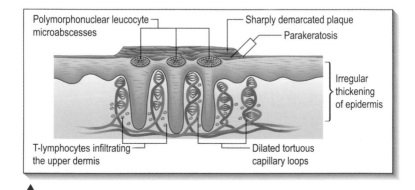

▲

Fig. 4.1 The changes seen in psoriatic skin.

Plaque psoriasis
In this common type the fully developed lesion is red, raised, clearly demarcated from the surrounding normal skin and has whitish scaling on the surface. There may be itching. Plaques frequently occur on or near the elbows, knees and the lower back. In the scalp, another common site, the presence of hair often results in a marked build-up of scaling, which can make the psoriasis feel lumpy. Scratching the surface will increase the amount of scaling seen.

Flexural psoriasis
In body folds such as the armpits, groins, genital area and near the anus, psoriasis tends not to be scaly but red and shiny. This is due to occlusion preventing drying out. Fissures may develop.

Guttate psoriasis
From the Latin for raindrop, guttate psoriasis is the abrupt onset of numerous small red scaly lesions, often in a widespread distribution. Guttate psoriasis often occurs in children and adolescents and is usually preceded by a streptococcal tonsillitis or sore throat. This pattern has a reasonable chance of getting better spontaneously over a few weeks or months.

Palms and soles
Psoriasis localized to these surfaces often has a very thick outer layer, may be less red and cracking is a prominent feature. It can be very difficult to diagnose without psoriasis elsewhere on the body as the edges are not well demarcated.

Scalp
This is frequently involved and, as with the rest of the skin, areas of scaling are noted on a background of normal skin. Scale can be prominent to the point of lumpiness which is obvious on palpation. Scalp margin psoriasis is common and hair loss is rarely seen.

4.7 Are there any more uncommon patterns?

Yes, there are a couple of rarer presentations which can be medical emergencies.

■ *Erythrodermic psoriasis*: Erythroderma means red skin, and is used to describe situations where the entire skin (or nearly all of it) becomes red, with some degree of scaling. There is loss of normal temperature regulation, with shivering and feeling hot, and yet the internal temperature can become abnormally low. This uncommon pattern can have many causes – for example, an irritant treatment, withdrawal of steroid therapy or a medicine which can aggravate psoriasis such as the antimalarial chloroquine. It can be a medical emergency with the risk of high output cardiac failure.

■ *Pustular psoriasis*: Pustular psoriasis of the palms and soles sometimes occurs in the absence of any other psoriasis. On a background of red skin, the pustules are green or yellow, becoming brown as they come to the surface and are shed as scales. Although they contain pus, they are sterile as this is just due to the accumulation of polymorphs. This type of psoriasis is often sore or painful and is regarded as separate from psoriasis by some dermatologists who refer to it as palmoplantar pustulosis.

Much less common is generalized pustular psoriasis. Like erythrodermic psoriasis, this may have a trigger (e.g. withdrawal of a steroid treatment). Large areas of tender red skin become covered in numerous pustules. There is usually fever and malaise. Generalized pustular psoriasis is a serious condition requiring hospital admission.

4.8 Does psoriasis affect the nails?

Nail changes are common and not always noticed; in some patients they may be the only way in which psoriasis is being expressed. Pitting – many small depressions in the surface of the nail – is characteristic of psoriasis. Also common is separation of the nail from the nailbed – known as onycholysis; this may be accompanied by a reddish-brown discolouration of the nailbed next to where the nail is separated (oil drop sign). Nails can also be thickened, crumbly and with accumulated debris beneath – but these changes are also found in other conditions (e.g. fungal infection).

4.9 What is psoriatic arthropathy?

As well as psoriasis, some patients have the added problem of a form of arthritis specific to psoriasis; this is termed psoriatic arthropathy. This is probably much more common than previously thought as one radiographic study showed specific joint changes in 50% of a group of psoriatic patients. Most of these were asymptomatic at the time so the true prevalence may be closer to 15%.

4.10 Are there different types of arthritis linked to psoriasis?

Psoriatic arthropathy can be classified into five different types so the answer is 'yes'! Although it is easy to note these classifications, real patients can present with features that cross the classifications or change with time.

■ *Asymmetrical oligoarthritis* – one or two large joints unilaterally. Around 70% of cases present like this but some progress on to symmetrical polyarthritis.

■ *Symmetrical polyarthritis* – affects both large and small joints. It accounts for 15% of cases and can be difficult to distinguish clinically from rheumatoid arthritis. Of patients with this form, 50% will experience relentless progression.

■ *Distal interphalangeal arthritis* – a well-recognized pattern in the hands and feet, especially in the presence of nail changes. Usually mild, chronic and not particularly disabling, it accounts for between 5 and 10% of cases.

■ *Spondylitis and enthesopathy* – similar to ankylosing spondylitis with sacroiliitis and inflammation around large tendon insertions.

■ *Arthritis mutilans* – a frightening term for the most severe form of psoriatic arthropathy. Gross deformity, subluxations and loss of bone from osteolysis can make this very disabling.

4.11 With psoriatic arthropathy, does the psoriasis rash on the skin appear at the same time as the arthritis?

It can do but it can also appear before or after. The majority of people (60%) will have the rash before the arthropathy, 15% will get both at the same time and 25% will get the joint problems first. It is worth asking about family history of psoriasis if you suspect psoriatic arthropathy without a rash and also examining the nails for supportive clues.

4.12 Is the incidence of psoriasis equal in both sexes?

Overall, yes, but there are some interesting differences in that men are more likely to get distal interphalangeal and spinal problems and women are more likely to get symmetrical polyarthropathy.

4.13 Is the incidence of arthropathy linked to the severity of the psoriasis?

This is difficult to evaluate as the severity of the psoriasis may vary over time. There does seem to be some link in that, if 15% is the overall incidence in patients with psoriasis, the incidence in those with severe psoriasis seems to be 25%.

4.14 What differential diagnoses are there for psoriasis?

Sometimes other skin diseases, as outlined in *Table 4.1*, can resemble psoriasis.

4.15 Are there any useful investigations in the diagnosis of psoriasis?

Sometimes tests are useful:

■ A skin biopsy to exclude a condition for which the treatment would be completely different

TABLE 4.1 Differential diagnosis in psoriasis

Condition	Like psoriasis	Unlike psoriasis
Discoid eczema	Red scaly itchy patches	Less well defined. Surface often blistering or crusted. Not usually in the same distribution
Seborrhoeic eczema	Involvement of scalp, armpits	Less well defined. More diffuse in scalp and groins/anogenital area
Fungal infection:		
Skin	Red scaly patches	Scaling mainly at the edge of lesions
Nails	Onycholysis, thickened and crumbly nails	No fine pits or oil drop sign
Pityriasis rosea	Small red scaly patches may resemble guttate psoriasis	Larger lesions are ovoid and have a ring of scale inside the outer border of each lesion. Less intensely red

- A swab to exclude bacterial infection
- A skin scraping or nail clipping to examine for fungal infection
- A throat swab if a bacterial throat infection may be triggering guttate psoriasis
- A trial with a treatment which only improves psoriasis – only helpful if the condition then improves.

4.16 What types of treatment are there?

Psoriasis can be successfully treated in most patients, but it must be emphasized that whatever is used is treatment for that episode, not a cure for the whole disease.

Before embarking on the details of treatments, it is essential to explore the patient's concerns about the disease. There may be fears based on the way psoriasis behaved in a relative or friend, concerns that psoriasis is catching or somehow related to cancer. Enquire about how the psoriasis impacts on the patient's work, leisure activities (many with psoriasis give up swimming etc.) and relationships.

There is no single treatment that is best for everyone and often different treatments are combined for maximal benefit. The choice depends on the type of psoriasis (plaque, guttate, pustular, erythrodermic), where it is on the body, how extensive it is, and how much trouble it is causing. Sometimes the choice may be limited by medical considerations.

Topical treatments

These can be used at home for localized areas of psoriasis and, in dermatology centres, treatments that would be impractical for home use can be applied by the nursing staff. An emollient, especially soft white paraffin, can improve minimal psoriasis, reducing scaling and sometimes other signs. This is perhaps the single most underused form of treatment for psoriasis. It can greatly improve a patient's comfort with reduction in itching and scaling. Active treatments for psoriasis include topical steroids, vitamin D analogues (calcipotriol, tacalcitol and calcitriol), tazarotene (a vitamin A derivative), coal tar preparations and dithranol. All these can be effective, at best clearing the psoriasis, sometimes with lengthy remissions before relapse occurs. All except the topical steroids can be irritant. The steroids are best used for short periods at a time, because of the risk of side effects such as skin thinning and the need for ever stronger preparations to maintain some benefit.

Ultraviolet radiation – 'light treatment'

Widespread psoriasis can be difficult and time consuming to treat with creams etc. For guttate psoriasis and for many patients with widespread plaque psoriasis, therapeutic ultraviolet (UV) radiation can be effective. Most hospital dermatology departments offer narrowband UVB. The combination of longer wave UVA with the plant derivative psoralen (PUVA) is also useful. UVB and UVA are described further in *Question 4.19*.

Systemic treatments

Several drugs have proved useful in controlling the most severe types of psoriasis. Some of these modify the body's immune system, reduce the rate at which cells divide, or do both; these include methotrexate, ciclosporin and hydroxycarbamide. Others have different actions – for example, acitretin (a vitamin A derivative) and fumaric acid esters.

Recently a number of new bioengineered drugs have appeared for psoriasis. These have highly specific actions and may have less likelihood for side effects. In the USA the following have proved effective: etanercept, infliximab, alefacept and efalizumab. At the time of writing only efalizumab has been licensed in the UK; they will all be very expensive and have not yet been reviewed by the National Institute for Clinical Excellence (NICE).

As with topical treatments, patients vary as to which systemic drug will suit them best. In the UK all the systemic drugs are supervised by a dermatologist although often the GP is involved with monitoring for side effects.

Treatment in hospital

For some types of psoriasis (e.g. erythrodermic or generalized pustular psoriasis) rest in hospital is a valuable element in management.

4.17 When should patients be referred to hospital?

As for eczema, NICE has produced guidelines for referral (*see Appendix*) which acknowledge that most patients can be managed in primary care. The reasons given for referral of patients to a specialist service are:

- they have generalized pustular or erythrodermic psoriasis
- their psoriasis is acutely unstable
- they have widespread symptomatic guttate psoriasis that would benefit from phototherapy
- the condition is causing severe social or psychological problems; prompts to referral should include sleeplessness, social exclusion, and reduced quality of life or self-esteem
- the rash is sufficiently extensive to make self-management impractical
- the rash is in a sensitive area (such as face, hands, feet, genitalia) and the symptoms particularly troublesome
- the rash is leading to time off work or school sufficient to interfere with employment or education
- they require assessment for the management of associated arthropathy
- the rash fails to respond to management in general practice. Failure is probably best based on the subjective assessment of the patient. Sometimes failure occurs when patients are unable to apply treatments themselves
- they have, or develop, features that make the diagnosis uncertain.

4.18 What is known about the use of inositol to counter the effect of lithium if patients cannot discontinue it?

Lithium is sometimes the only effective drug for patients with bipolar affective disorders, but it often makes psoriasis worse. Inositol depletion occurs during lithium therapy and may explain some of the drug's side effects. Giving inositol supplements (6 g/day) has been shown to improve psoriasis in patients on lithium in one well-conducted, double-blind, placebo-controlled trial (*see Bibliography, Allan et al 2004*).

4.19 How safe is ultraviolet treatment?

Both UVB and PUVA can produce unpleasant side effects at the time the radiation is given, and PUVA can cause both skin cancer and photoageing in the long term (*see Fig. 5.2*). Nevertheless, if used appropriately, both are valuable treatments, particularly if the psoriasis is widespread.

The main short-term side effect of UVB is burning, similar to sunburn. This is less likely to occur with the more modern narrowband UVB. Broadband UVB has been in use for more than 70 years, and in most studies there is no increased risk of skin cancer except on the male genital skin when high doses were used. Narrowband UVB has not been in use long enough for its long-term consequences to be known.

PUVA, the combination of the photosensitizing drug psoralen and longer wavelength UVA, has been widely used for the past 30 years. Like UVB, PUVA can produce changes resembling sunburn. During treatment, other side effects experienced include tanning, pruritus (itching) and occasionally pain. When psoralen is given by mouth, nausea can occur. Nowadays PUVA is given in courses rather than continuously. The long-term risks of PUVA mainly occur in those who burn easily and do not readily tan. After many treatments, dark irregularly-shaped freckles and at least some degree of so-called ageing changes as occur after many years of sun exposure are common. The risk of skin cancer is increased, especially for squamous cell carcinoma.

4.20 Do systemic treatments need monitoring?

All the treatments for psoriasis given by mouth or injection can have unwanted effects, and the objective of monitoring is to recognize an event that might be serious before it has become so.

Monitoring is usually a shared activity. The person with psoriasis should be aware of symptoms that might mean the systemic treatment should be adjusted or even stopped. The general practice is likely to be involved with routine blood tests and for ciclosporin measurement of blood pressure; the dermatologist will be responsible for other aspects such as liver biopsy and specialized blood tests (*Table 4.2*), and for overall supervision. With most

---

TABLE 4.2 Common drug monitoring tests

Drug	Event being monitored	Test
Methotrexate	Bone marrow suppression	Full blood count
	Liver abnormalities	Routine liver tests
		Procollagen peptide*
		Liver biopsy*
Ciclosporin	Hypertension	Blood pressure
	Kidney impairment	Creatinine, urea, electrolytes
Acitretin	Fat metabolism	Cholesterol, triglycerides
	Liver abnormalities	Routine liver tests
Hydroxycarbamide	Bone marrow suppression	Full blood count

*These tests are carried out under the supervision of a dermatologist

drugs, monitoring is carried out more intensively early on and when the dosage is increased.

4.21 Are there likely to be any new developments in management?

Several bioengineered treatments have been evaluated for psoriasis during the past few years. Each blocks a particular element of the several events that contribute to the formation of psoriasis. In this respect the action is more specific than the existing systemic drugs. The new treatments are all given by injection, for the more severe end of the psoriasis spectrum. Those most studied are efalizumab, etanercept, infliximab and alefacept. Efalizumab and etanercept are now available in the UK for psoriasis; infliximab has recently been used here for rheumatoid arthritis and some other chronic inflammatory diseases including 'off label' treatment of psoriasis.

These new treatments appear promising, sometimes with benefit lasting well beyond the course of injections. None of the new agents has proved to be very successful in more than about two-thirds of the patients treated. Whether there will be longer term side effects that have not occurred during the time the drugs have been in use remains to be seen.

All of these treatments are very expensive.

4.22 Are there any psychological treatments that can help?

Patients can become very upset by having psoriasis and also find that stressful events in their lives can make the psoriasis worse. It is possible for this to lead to a downward spiral, leaving a very depressed and demotivated person with bad psoriasis. Good support, empathy and allowing patients time to talk about how they feel about their skin and themselves can help but more specific therapies have recently been shown to be of real benefit. Surveys carried out by patient support groups have shown that 60% of patients believe that stress is a trigger for their psoriasis so much more research needs to be carried out into ways of addressing this.

One of the problems for patients with psoriasis seems to be stigmatization. This applies to many disfiguring skin problems but seems to be much more of a problem in psoriasis and can persist, even after successful treatment to clear the skin. If patients have a fear of stigmatization, this limits their social interaction and lessens the chance of them receiving positive feedback from people who don't respond negatively to the skin problem. It is also known that psychological factors can limit the response to physical treatments such as PUVA and may influence compliance with other treatment regimens, with up to 40% of patients admitting that they do not adhere to treatment advice.

Cognitive behavioural therapy is a psychological approach that looks at thought processes and, in psoriasis, can help to:

- modify inaccurate and unhelpful beliefs
- modify ineffective coping behaviour
- modify negative mood states.

Recent research has shown a significant and ongoing benefit lasting for 6 months after only six sessions of therapy. It is not yet widely available but should become more so, especially as its role in treating depression is also becoming recognized.

This alleviation of anxiety and a better response to treatment, combined with a better understanding of the disease, seems to allow patients to achieve emotional distance from their skin problems and become more self-motivated. In this state of mind, they develop a sense of control over the psoriasis. Since this sense of control needs to be realistic, it also involves discussion between clinician and patient to make sure that expectations of treatment and progress match up.

 PATIENT QUESTIONS

4.23 Is psoriasis linked to hormonal changes?

There is no clear evidence about this but some women certainly report variation in their disease with monthly cycles. In most pregnancies, the psoriasis also varies – it usually improves but can get worse in some cases. The fact that the two main peaks of onset of psoriasis are around the time of puberty and the menopause does suggest some hormonal trigger at work but no studies have ever suggested that a hormonal treatment could work.

4.24 Should I buy a sunbed?

No. UV light can lead to the development of skin cancers and needs to be properly controlled and the cumulative dose monitored carefully. If your psoriasis gets better in the sun you should discuss a referral for treatment.

4.25 I have had one episode of guttate psoriasis – will I go on to get plaque psoriasis?

Guttate psoriasis may be the first ever presentation but can also occur in patients who have established psoriasis. The chance of developing plaque psoriasis is probably raised compared to someone who has never had guttate psoriasis but it is difficult to put this any more definitively.

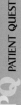

4.26   Do I have to treat all my psoriasis?

No, it is your skin and your psoriasis. Leaving some areas untreated will make no difference to the overall progress of the problem. Many people concentrate on the visible parts of the body, using active treatments on the face and hands, whilst just using a moisturizer to keep other areas as comfortable as possible. It is always worth using a moisturizer even if you don't want to actively treat all the plaques.

Skin reactions to light

5

5.1   What is ultraviolet light?

We tend to use the term 'light' for that part of the electromagnetic spectrum which we can see; the rest (e.g. x-rays, gamma rays, microwaves and infra red) we term radiation (*Fig. 5.1*). Ultraviolet is invisible to us, although it can be perceived by some living creatures, so is better termed ultraviolet radiation (abbreviated here to UV).

UV is divided into C, B and A – C being the segment with the shortest wavelength; UVC is absorbed by ozone in the atmosphere so does not reach the earth's surface.

5.2   What effect does ultraviolet light have on the skin?

UVB includes the wavelengths which cause redness, sunburn, skin cancer and some of the changes associated with ageing (*Fig. 5.2*). Very little UVB penetrates below the level of the epidermis. The longer wavelength UVA stimulates the pigment cells (melanocytes) to produce melanin, but does not cause sunburn. It penetrates deeper into the skin than UVB. It contributes to skin ageing and skin cancer as it is capable of damaging DNA. Some of the allergic reactions to drugs in which UV plays a part are due to UVA wavelengths.

5.3   Does it matter what colour the skin is?

Melanin, the complex pigment produced by the melanocytes, has the ability to absorb UVB. Generally speaking, the more natural pigment a person has the less harmful exposure to UV will be. For example, skin

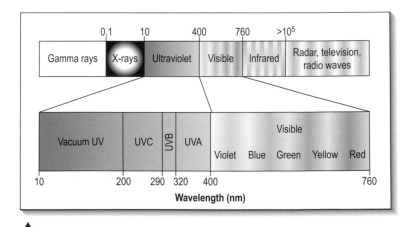

▲

Fig. 5.1 The electromagnetic spectrum and ultraviolet radiation.

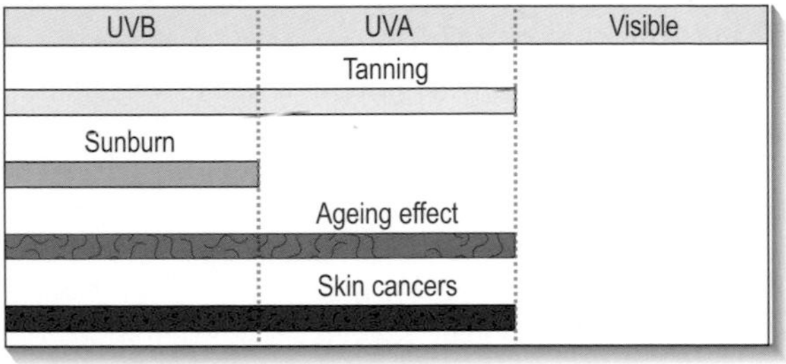

▲

Fig. 5.2 Effects of different wavelengths of light on the skin.

cancer due to sun exposure is rare in those with so-called black skin. Unfortunately getting a tan is not a recommended form of sun protection for those with lighter skin. Skin is classified into several grades (*Table 5.1*).

5.4   How should sunburn be managed?

Sunburn is a consequence of sufficient UVB interacting with substances in the epidermal cells leading to the release of molecules which cause inflammation. The skin becomes red several hours later, and in severe cases, blistering can occur (*see Ch. 9*). If the burn is extensive and severe, there will be loss of fluid and pain. The consequences are similar to other types of burn, and treatment of severe sunburn should be at a burns unit. Lesser degrees of sunburn can be helped in terms of the symptoms by bland soothing preparations such as oily calamine lotion. It has been suggested that early use of a topical steroid is useful. Aspirin may be an effective painkiller. Despite sunburn being very common, there is little good scientific work to guide us as to the best treatment for the less severe case. It is always worth taking the opportunity to emphasize the need for avoiding excessive exposure.

TABLE 5.1 Skin – a classification by grade

Grade	Effect of UVB	Skin type
1	Always burns but never tans	Pale skin, red hair, freckles
2	Usually burns, sometimes tans	Fair skin
3	May burn, usually tans	Darker skin
4	Rarely burns, always tans	Pale brown
5	Rarely burns, tans profusely	Dark brown
6	Never burns	'Black', i.e. very dark brown

5.5 What is phototoxicity?

Phototoxicity resembles sunburn but is due to a reaction between sunlight and a drug taken by mouth or a chemical absorbed into the skin from contact (e.g. certain plants). Phototoxicity comes on quickly after exposure to UV and when the inflammation has settled down it is often followed by darkening of the skin. Such reactions can occur due to UVA as well as UVB, so can be triggered by exposure in a tanning salon. Phototoxicity does not involve the immune system. Allergic reactions in which UV plays a part do occur (photoallergy), but more commonly produce a reaction like contact eczema (*see Q 2.4*).

Some drugs are much more likely to produce phototoxic reactions (e.g. amiodarone); with others the individual risk is small, but many cases do occur because the drug is very widely used (e.g. thiazides) (*Box 5.1*).

5.6 How does phototoxicity present?

Most phototoxicity reactions resemble sunburn and occur quickly after exposure to UV. There will be redness, discomfort and, in severe cases, blistering on the sun-exposed skin. When due to a drug, any sun-exposed areas can be affected; if there has been contact with the phototoxic substance (e.g. from rubbing against a plant), the phototoxic rash will usually be where there has been both contact and exposure to UV. After the acute reaction has settled down there is often an increase in skin pigmentation.

BOX 5.1 Substances producing phototoxic reactions

Drugs
- Amiodarone
- Thiazides
- Non-steroidal anti-inflammatory drugs
- Phenothiazines, e.g. chlorpromazine
- Sulphonamides, e.g. co-trimoxazole
- Fluoroquinolones, e.g. ciprofloxacin
- Tetracyclines, e.g. doxycycline
- Psoralens (as used in PUVA)
- Chlorpropamide

Contact substances
- Tar
- Psoralens in plants

5.7 Is phototoxicity just an acute reaction or can it be a chronic reaction?

Occasionally inflammation generated by exposure to sunlight continues long term. The skin will be red, thickened, and may resemble eczema. Changes occur on light-exposed sites such as the forehead, nose, cheeks, chin, backs of the hands and lower front of the neck. This may occur when the body's immune system is responsible for the reaction. Photoallergic reactions can occur with some drugs (e.g. the sulphonamides); other causes include certain plants (e.g. chrysanthemums). Just as patch tests (*see Q 2.29*) can help determine the cause of contact eczema, a modification (photo patch tests) can be used to identify possible causes in such cases. Some patients with atopic eczema have chronic photosensitivity. Particularly in elderly men, chronic UV reactions can be severe and difficult to prevent with sunscreens.

5.8 What is 'strimmer dermatitis'?

This is a phrase coined to suit patients admitted with widespread phyto-phototoxic reactions after using a strimmer to clear weeds in the garden. Patients were mainly men who had been working in the sun wearing only a pair of shorts. The action of the strimmer threw up droplets of plant juices leading to the widespread blistering eruption which often merited admission.

5.9 What is 'sun allergy'?

After sunburn the commonest skin condition occurring after sun exposure to UV is polymorphic light eruption (PLE) – variously known as sun allergy and heat rash (and wrongly as prickly heat: this is due to heat, not UV, and involves the sweat glands).

PLE mainly affects young women. It is termed polymorphic because of the variety of appearances: there are usually itchy red papules affecting only the sun-exposed areas, but blistering and oedema can also occur. The condition usually comes on between several hours to a few days after sun exposure and typically begins in the spring but gradually subsides before summer ends. PLE can often be avoided with common-sense measures – for example, avoiding the sun at its most intense, appropriate clothing and broad-spectrum sunscreens. Some cases respond to topical steroids. Courses of PUVA or narrowband UVB given before the expected onset can provide effective prophylaxis. Hydroxychloroquine can be effective, beta carotene is occasionally used, and, if all else fails, oral steroids will usually help.

5.10 Is polymorphic light eruption the same as actinic prurigo?

No. Actinic prurigo is a much less common condition, mainly beginning in childhood. It is less obviously sunshine related; although worse in summer and on light-exposed skin, it can persist in winter and occur on light-protected skin. Like PLE, actinic prurigo is itchy, and the appearance is of scratched spots and lumps.

Most patients have an uncommon HLA-DR haplotype, implying that there is a genetic basis.

5.11 What about skin cancer?

The commonest skin cancers are basal cell carcinoma, squamous cell carcinoma and malignant melanoma (*see Ch. 12*). Most of these are due to previous sun exposure. Sometimes this is obvious, in that the cancer occurs on the most sun-exposed parts. Episodes of burn may be at least as important as repeated exposure. Those protected by naturally dark skin are the least likely to get these skin cancers (*see Q 5.3*).

5.12 Are any skin diseases helped by the sun?

The UV component of sunlight often improves psoriasis, sometimes eczema, and a few other uncommon skin conditions – for example, pityriasis lichenoides, parapsoriasis and the itch of some internal disorders such as chronic liver disease and kidney failure. It is not good practice to advise patients to use sunlight or sunbeds to treat their skin as the exposure to UV is not controlled and monitored so they could be at increased risk of skin cancer. Those who report benefit could be referred to a specialist for UV therapy.

5.13 Does sunlight make any diseases worse?

Apart from the phototoxic reactions described already, probably the commonest skin disease to be triggered by sun exposure is an outbreak of herpes simplex (cold sore) on or near the lips. Lupus erythematosus (LE) (*see Ch. 8*) – both the purely cutaneous and systemic types – can be worsened or brought on by the sun. In some people the sun makes psoriasis and eczema worse rather than better. Some rarer diseases aggravated by sun exposure include most of the porphyrias, Darier's disease, the vitamin B_6 deficiency state pellagra and the diseases in which there is an inherited defect in repairing UV-induced damage to DNA such as xeroderma pigmentosum (*see Q 12.7*).

5.14 Is skin ageing caused by long-term sun exposure?

Compare the skin on the face and the back of the hand of someone aged 60 with the skin under the chin of the same person and you will see that much of what we regard as ageing is due to the cumulative effects of sun exposure.

Sun damage shows as wrinkling, thickened yellowish areas, bruising after minor knocks and brown blotches. Pick up a fold of skin and let go – the sun-damaged skin will have poor recoil due to changes in the connective tissue. Feel the surface – there may be rough patches suggesting actinic keratoses.

Age alone does produce changes in all the skin – for example, the dermis becomes thinner and loses some of its resilience. Nonetheless, skin protected from UV will look and feel much 'younger' than exposed skin.

 PATIENT QUESTIONS

5.15 What is prickly heat?

This has the more medical name of miliaria rubra and is to do with heat, not UV radiation. The sweat glands become blocked so sweat is retained within the skin producing itchy bumps and sometimes small blisters. It represents a failure to adapt to hot climates so can improve as you get used to the heat. Treatment is to get out of the heat, preferably to a cool air-conditioned room. Mild steroids such as hydrocortisone can help relieve the symptoms.

5.16 What is the best way to protect my skin from the sun?

The best way is to avoid going out in the sun! As this may be very difficult and there are well-recognized psychological benefits from being in the sun, especially on holiday, there are several key things to remember. The sun is at its strongest around the middle of the day so try to avoid it between 11 a.m. and 3 p.m. Stick to the shade and wear clothing thick enough or coloured enough to give protection from UV – thin, light-coloured T-shirts are not very good at blocking UV. Beware of reflected UV from white walls, pavements and the sea. Wear a broad-brimmed hat and sunglasses. Last of all, use a good sunscreen and reapply it frequently, especially if you are in and out of the sea or sweating a lot.

5.17 Are all sunscreens the same?

No, sunscreens vary in their ability to block UV and also whether they block just UVB or UVA as well. The packaging may give an indication of the SPF and a star rating. SPF stands for sun protection factor but is really only a measure of UVB blocking; the higher the SPF the better, especially for children or those with sensitive, fair skin. An SPF of 15 means that you could stay in the sun for 15 hours to get the same exposure as you would in 1 hour without it. It has to be realized that this is only if the sunscreen works at its best for the whole 15 hours! Repeated application would be necessary to achieve this in real life. One of the problems with UVB blocking is that it prevents the burning effect and can lead to longer exposure to UVA which causes deep-down damage. The star rating system is a measure of the effectiveness of UVA block. Always remember that a sunscreen is the last resort if you cannot avoid the sun; keep to the shade or wear protective clothes and a hat.

Bacterial and viral infections

6

6.1 How common are infections of the skin?

Disease due to microorganisms in or on the skin is part of the human experience. Although defences against pathogenic bacteria, fungi, viruses and protozoa are generally very effective, infections are inevitable, and some are very common. Most people at some stage will experience viral warts, tinea pedis, impetigo and folliculitis.

6.2 Why are skin infections important?

Changes in the skin are often the clue that a patient has a potentially serious systemic infection – for example, secondary syphilis, the characteristic lesions of meningococcal septicaemia and leprosy. Infections of the skin are often self-limiting and have little impact, but can be important for one or more of the following reasons: if they

- *become systemic* – either by direct invasion (e.g. septicaemia from cellulitis, herpes encephalitis from eczema herpeticum) or liberation of a toxin which enters the circulation (e.g. staphylococcal scalded skin (*see Q 6.11*) and toxic shock syndromes).
- *cause a severe inflammatory reaction* – sometimes the reaction to a minor infection is serious (e.g. recurrent Stevens–Johnson syndrome due to herpes simplex).
- *cause significant morbidity* – skin infections can cause permanent destructive changes (e.g. severe scalp fungal infection can cause irreversible hair loss, leishmaniasis often produces disfigurement). Even when not destructive, skin infections can cause functional impairment, at times for long periods (e.g. painful plantar warts). Psychological consequences of skin infection should not be ignored: diseases that are medically trivial like pityriasis versicolor can interfere with self-esteem more than is often recognized.
- *be a clue to serious internal disease* – unusually extensive or severe manifestations of some skin infections may be the clue that a patient has immunodeficiency (e.g. widespread molluscum contagiosum in an adult can be an initial manifestation of AIDS).

BACTERIAL INFECTIONS

6.3 What is the most common bacterial infection of the skin?

In children, impetigo is common. It is usually recognizable by the presence of fragile clear or turbid fluid-filled blisters on a red base, often breaking to give crusted erosions. Lesions spread quickly, and to those in close contact. Eczema is often complicated by impetigo. Impetigo is usually caused by

Staphylococcus aureus, although *Streptococcus pyogenes* can be present either alone or in combination.

In older people, staphylococcal infection of hair follicles is the commonest manifestation, producing boils (folliculitis or furunculosis) (*Fig. 6.1*).

6.4 Is staphylococcus the most common cause of bacterial skin infection?

By causing most cases of furunculosis and impetigo, *Staphylococcus aureus* is the commonest cause of bacterial infection of the skin.

Other important bacterial pathogens are beta haemolytic streptococci (causing erysipelas, some cellulitis and necrotizing fasciitis), mycobacteria (tuberculosis, leprosy), spirochaetes (syphilis, Lyme disease) and many others including anthrax.

6.5 What is folliculitis?

Folliculitis is inflammation of the hair follicle. When the inflammation is deep the term furunculosis is often used. Not all folliculitis is due to infection – examples of non-infective folliculitis include the sterile follicular pustules which can occur from contact with oil and other chemicals and after epilation (plucking out hairs). Although *Staphylococcus aureus* is a common infective cause, other microbes can cause folliculitis – for example, the Malassezia yeasts in seborrhoeic folliculitis, dermatophyte fungi (especially in tinea inadvertently treated with topical steroids) and Gram-negative folliculitis in antibiotic-treated acne. Furunculosis is a destructive process and the lesions begin as follicular nodules. These are usually due to *Staphylococcus aureus*.

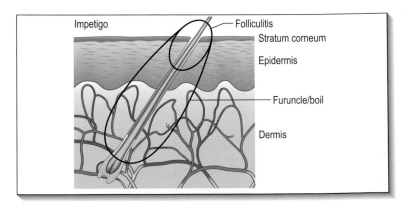

▲

Fig. 6.1 Schematic showing the depths of different bacterial infections of the skin.

6.6   Can you catch folliculitis from a Jacuzzi?

You can certainly catch an infection which causes folliculitis from Jacuzzis and hot tubs. If the water becomes contaminated with Pseudomonas there is a significant risk for all users to develop a rash. This usually erupts about 48 hours after exposure with a range of 8 hours to 5 days. The rash takes the form of multiple pruritic papules, pustules or vesicles, or sometimes all three, with surrounding urticaria. It lasts 7–10 days but can be recurrent even without further exposure. Simple emollients and antiseptics may help but if the rash doesn't seem to be clearing, ciprofloxacin should treat the Pseudomonas.

6.7   What is the best way to manage superficial skin infections such as impetigo and furunculosis?

Localized impetigo responds well to topical agents. Impetigo is due to either *Staphylococcus aureus* or *Streptococcus pyogenes* or both. Topical mupirocin and fusidic acid are both highly effective, but remember that the latter is also used systemically and resistance can be a real problem. Resistance is more likely if it is used for lengthy periods or repeatedly – as could happen in eczema sufferers – and community-acquired staphylococci are increasingly resistant to it. Neomycin is effective against staphylococci but less so against streptococci. Bacitracin is effective against both. If there are thick crusts, gentle removal is worthwhile before using any topical agent.

If impetigo is widespread, or if there is lymphadenopathy and/or fever, then an oral antibiotic should be used. Flucloxacillin is generally the first choice with erythromycin as an alternative for penicillin-allergic patients, although there can be local resistance to the latter. It is always worth checking with your local microbiologist for advice.

Infection of hair follicles is called folliculitis if superficial and furunculosis (boils) if deep. For widespread cases of either, flucloxacillin or another penicillinase-resistant agent should be used. If the condition is recurrent, exclude diabetes and swab the nose and perineum for evidence of carriage in the patient and other members of the household.

6.8   Are cellulitis and erysipelas the same?

Erysipelas is an acute bacterial infection of the dermis and perhaps the upper subcutaneous fat, typically due to *Streptococcus pyogenes*. Cellulitis is inflammation of the subcutaneous tissues, often due to *Streptococcus pyogenes*, but can also be caused by other bacteria, occasionally deep fungi and non-infective causes.

In both conditions there is redness, tenderness, swelling and warmth; because erysipelas is more superficial there is a better defined edge, which is often palpable. Because erysipelas can extend deeply and cellulitis superficially, the two processes do overlap. Classical erysipelas is, however, a recognizable disease – and nearly always due to beta haemolytic streptococci.

6.9 Should cellulitis and erysipelas always be treated in hospital? If not, what should the approach be in primary care?

There will be many circumstances when it is reasonable to initiate treatment in primary care for limited areas of cellulitis or erysipelas. Treatment should be with amoxicillin 500 mg 8 hourly plus flucloxacillin 500 mg 6 hourly for an adult who is not allergic to penicillins. If allergic, either clarithromycin 250 mg b.d. or clindamycin 150 mg 6 hourly should be satisfactory. It is essential that the patient is reviewed after 24 hours. If there is no improvement, the patient should be transferred to secondary care with a view to having parenteral treatment. If there is improvement, continue treatment for at least 7 days.

The situations where it is best to refer immediately to hospital are if the cellulitis/erysipelas:

- is extensive
- is very painful
- is purpuric and/or fluctuant
- involves the orbit
- is associated with a penetrating injury or bite
- is in a limb which is post-phlebitic, lymphoedematous or arterially impaired.

The patient's overall health also merits consideration – for example, if the patient:

- is septic and hypotensive
- is diabetic
- is immunocompromised
- has varicella
- has sickle cell disease
- is an infant or very old
- is an intravenous drug user.

6.10 Why is necrotizing fasciitis serious?

Necrotizing fasciitis is one of a group of subcutaneous infections in which necrosis occurs, there is severe toxicity and appreciable mortality. Necrotizing fasciitis is usually due to group A streptococci although other organisms can be involved. The initial presentation is like cellulitis, with a hot, red, tender swelling. The pain is excruciating and out of all proportion to the initial presentation. Bullae and necrosis then occur. Antibiotics alone cannot control the process, and surgical removal of all necrotic tissue is essential. Urgent admission is essential to avoid massive tissue loss with the risk of fatality.

6.11 What is scalded skin syndrome?

Staphylococcal scalded skin syndrome is due to the effects of a blood-borne toxin. There is usually only a trivial focus of infection (e.g. a stye). Typically the patient is a young child who becomes febrile, irritable, and has spreading redness and tenderness of the skin, soon followed by superficial blistering. There can be large areas of loss of the outer part of the epidermis. The disease is painful and requires hospital admission. Staphylococcal scalded skin syndrome can occur rarely in older patients, but there is usually a predisposing factor such as renal failure or immunosuppression.

6.12 Is toxic epidermal necrolysis the same as scalded skin syndrome?

No. The depth of tissue loss is greater in toxic epidermal necrolysis as the full thickness of the epidermis is lost, not just the stratum corneum, and mucosal surfaces are affected. This is usually a drug reaction so is nothing to do with infection. Urgent admission is needed to prevent life-threatening infection and to replace lost fluids and electrolytes as for extensive burns.

6.13 What is fish-tank granuloma?

Fish-tank granuloma is a chronic skin infection with *Mycobacterium marinum*. This environmental mycobacterium is found in water (salty and fresh) in natural lakes and seas and artificial enclosures. The commonest source nowadays is in tropical fish tanks where it causes an ultimately fatal infection in the fish. Entry of the bacterium in humans is usually through a minor abrasion – often on the hand. After an incubation period that can last many weeks, the lesion grows to form a verrucous plaque, nodule or, sometimes, ulcer. A characteristic feature is the occurrence of new nodules along the course of the lymphatics. The disease usually remains confined to one limb and is diagnosed by histology and culture of part of a lesion. The lesions can heal very slowly but patients usually prefer treatment with minocycline 100 mg b.d. for 6–12 weeks. Patients should be advised to use rubber gloves when cleaning out their tropical fish tanks or removing dead fish in the future.

6.14 Is Lyme disease an infection?

Lyme disease, named after a town in Connecticut where the disease made its first appearance in the USA in the 1970s, is caused by the spirochaete *Borrelia burgdorferi*. It is transmitted by ticks that normally feed on deer and sheep. After the bite, the characteristic lesion erythema chronicum migrans develops. This is an outwardly spreading red ring that evolves over a few weeks. The organism replicates in this skin lesion. At this time, some general symptoms such as headache, low grade fever, fatigue and muscle aches are quite common. Less commonly, meningitis, cranial nerve palsies and cardiac symptoms can occur. Chronic manifestations coming on months or years after the initial infection and analogous to late syphilis include arthritis and various central and peripheral nervous system problems.

Diagnosis is usually by serology. This can be negative early in the course of the disease, in which case specialized tests such as western blot are used.

6.15 How should Lyme disease be treated?

Early disease, with erythema chronicum migrans and mild constitutional symptoms, can be treated with amoxicillin 500 mg t.d.s. or doxycycline 100 mg b.d. for 14–21 days. Patients with significant neurological, cardiac or joint disease should be referred to secondary care.

6.16 If there ever was an outbreak of anthrax, what would the skin lesions look like?

The most striking thing about a typical anthrax lesion is the degree and extent of surrounding oedema. The initial lesion is a papule which develops into a blister or pustule on an oedematous base. Blisters break, forming a haemorrhagic crust around which further blisters develop. Despite the marked oedema, there is little or no lymphadenopathy. Images can be viewed on the internet at www.lib.uiowa.edu/hardin/md/dermpictures.html.

6.17 What is the best treatment for bacterial infection?

Usually it is best to know what bacteria are causing the infection and, if resistance might be a problem, choose an agent to which the organism is sensitive and will kill the bacteria quickly. Sometimes for skin infections it is reasonable to use topical treatment (e.g. mupirocin for impetigo). It never does any harm to take samples for bacterial culture and sensitivities, and these are very useful if the first choice of treatment proves unsuccessful. It is worth discussing this question with a local microbiologist who will know the local sensitivities and resistance problems for the common infections.

6.18 Is there a need for any investigations?

For cases of minor localized staphylococcal infection it is reasonable not to investigate and use a topical antibiotic. If there is widespread impetigo, empirical treatment has failed, there is furunculosis or the clinical picture is unusual, then swab for culture and sensitivities. With suspected cellulitis or erysipelas, swabs are rarely helpful, but blood culture can be positive.

Sometimes it is appropriate to obtain a sample of tissue for culture. Serological tests (ASOT and ADB) can be useful for groups A, C and G streptococcal infection but may take a few days from the onset of symptoms to become positive.

Neutrophil leucocytosis and elevation of C-reactive protein are helpful supporting evidence for soft tissue infection such as cellulitis, especially if it is not clear whether an acute red tender swelling is cellulitis or some other pathological process.

6.19 How can recurrent infection be prevented?

There may be an underlying treatable dermatosis increasing susceptibility – for example, atopic eczema predisposing to recurrent staphylococcal infection. A patient with recurrent furunculosis should be evaluated at least for diabetes mellitus, and if suffering from other infections, for an immunological deficiency. Sometimes patients become reinfected with staphylococci from sites of asymptomatic carriage – the nose, axillae, perineum and toe clefts – so swabs from these areas (and the same sites in close family members), with appropriate treatment using topical measures, can prove helpful. Antiseptic washes can be used for skin sites and a topical antibiotic for the anterior nares.

Cellulitis can become a recurrent problem, especially when there is lymphoedema, and the cause in this situation is usually group A *Streptococcus pyogenes*. Further attacks can usually be prevented with prophylactic penicillin V 250–500 mg b.d. Recurrent attacks of cellulitis on the legs, especially in older patients, should raise the suspicion of an untreated portal of infection. This can often be from a chronic fungal infection of the toenails and surrounding skin and secondary bacterial colonization.

VIRAL INFECTIONS

6.20 What is orf and how should it be treated?

Orf is primarily a disease of young sheep and goats. It is caused by a parapox virus, distantly related to smallpox and molluscum contagiosum viruses. Human lesions are most common on the hands, forearms and face. After an incubation period of 5–6 days, the lesion begins as a papule. This soon becomes oedematous and either pustular or bullous, often with haemorrhage into it. The centre crusts over, is surrounded by a greyish or violaceous zone and then a ring of erythema. There may be mild constitutional upset. Lesions resolve without scarring after a few weeks so most cases do not need any treatment. Some persistent cases have been treated with cidofovir. Secondary bacterial infection can occur and should be treated appropriately.

6.21 Is there a best way to treat viral warts?

Consider the following observations:

- Viral warts will usually resolve eventually in most people with a normal immune system.
- There is no treatment that selectively and painlessly kills just the causative human papilloma virus. It can, for example, survive in liquid nitrogen at $-196.4°C$.
- Most of the current treatments cause tissue damage in an effort to get the immune system to recognize the presence of the virus.

If treatments are to be used there needs to be a justification for any nuisance value, and pain or other unpleasant consequences of the treatment such as depigmentation following cryotherapy.

For troublesome warts on the hands or feet, salicylic acid paint together with regular paring will have a high success rate if used diligently for up to 3 months. Liquid nitrogen cryotherapy is only marginally more successful; it is painful, but may be quicker. For anogenital warts topical podophyllotoxin and imiquimod can be used at home; cryotherapy and sometimes other destructive methods may be used in the hospital. Facial warts are probably best treated by careful cryotherapy or electrosurgery.

Other methods for treating warts are sometimes used by specialists in hospital departments but all have one or more drawbacks. Imiquimod is not licensed in the UK for the treatment of warts other than on the genital area, but is more widely used in other parts of the world.

6.22 How common is molluscum contagiosum?

This pox virus infection is common, particularly in children. There are no reliable figures as to exactly how common.

6.23 Does molluscum contagiosum require treatment?

Molluscum contagiosum is purely a skin disease, although in some cases, especially the immunosuppressed, it can be very widespread. As with warts, there is no specific antiviral agent. In those with a normal immune system the condition usually resolves in about 9 months but can sometimes take years. In the person who is old enough to want treatment, any of the various methods used can be considered. In the younger child it is usually best to wait for natural resolution. Many treatments have been advocated, including nitrogen and pricking the lesions with a sharpened wooden stick.

Imiquimod three times weekly looks promising, but is not yet licensed for this use and is very expensive. One cheaper approach recommended by some dermatologists is to apply 12% salicylic acid gel once a week and emollients on the days in between.

6.24 Is there a way to prevent recurrent attacks of herpes simplex?

Sometimes there are recognizable triggers for recurrences of herpes simplex (e.g. minor trauma and febrile illnesses).

Alas, these attacks are not generally treatable or predictable. Occasionally the trigger can be ameliorated – for example, the effects of sun exposure which can sometimes be blocked with use of a sunscreen. If attacks are frequent, prophylactic aciclovir 200–400 mg b.d. can be an effective preventive measure. It often needs to be taken long term.

6.25 What is hand, foot and mouth disease?

This is a distinctive viral infection, mainly caused by particular strains of Coxsackie virus. It is highly contagious and typically occurs in children but can occur in adults. After an incubation period of 3–6 days, there is a brief prodrome which can include mild fever, malaise, sore mouth, abdominal pain and cough, before lesions appear in the mouth and on the hands and feet.

The oral lesions begin as red macules, and evolve through vesicles to ulcers which can be painful. They can be on the tongue, buccal mucosa and palate. The skin lesions are on the sides of digits and the palmar/plantar surfaces. The fully developed lesions are distinctive ovoid grey blisters with a surrounding rim of bright red erythema and are orientated with the long axes along skin lines. The acral lesions usually last 5–10 days, heal without scarring and recurrences are unusual.

6.26 Are bacterial and viral infections more common if the patient has a chronic skin disease like eczema?

The patient with atopic eczema very often has *Staphylococcus aureus* and to a lesser extent *Streptococcus pyogenes* colonizing the eczematous skin. Some explanations for this include the following:

■ The bacteria seem to adhere better to the horny layer cells, and there is underproduction of antimicrobial peptides (an important non-immunological skin defence against microorganisms).

■ Actual infection with these bacteria is common, and in addition the bacteria can aggravate the eczema.

■ Another infection which can be different in those with atopic eczema is herpes simplex – which can be disseminated and sometimes involve internal organs (eczema herpeticum).

■ Atopics often have widespread outbreaks of viral warts and molluscum contagiosum.

■ Bacterial colonization of other types of eczema can occur but is less noticeable and is not a feature of psoriasis and most other skin diseases with an intact skin surface.

6.27 Are skin infections more common in patients with HIV and other problems involving the immune system?

Yes. However, skin infections are not an uncommon finding in immunocompetent patients. The difficulty is distinguishing when an infection is related to an underlying immune deficiency. However, there are some helpful pointers.

The infection is with a common pathogen but in an atypical pattern, site, distribution or presentation

Common examples of this would include molluscum contagiosum. In human immunodeficiency virus (HIV) infection this is found on the face and the lesions are smaller, flatter, more resistant to treatment and occur in adults. In contrast, in patients with a normal immune system, molluscum contagiosum occurs as a childhood infection, on the trunk and the lesions are large and protuberant. Generalized or extensive herpes simplex (excluding eczema herpeticum) and herpes zoster with a multidermatomal distribution would be other examples.

The infection is with an uncommon pathogen

Kaposi's sarcoma is now known to result from an infection with the human herpes virus 8. It is most commonly found in association with HIV and therefore indicative of the need to exclude this. Some of the atypical mycobacteria do not commonly cause cutaneous infection but may be found in the context of HIV.

The infection is persistent or recurrent even with treatment

Viral warts are a common infection. Their persistence, and widespread distribution, may be an indicator of an immunosuppressed patient. Furthermore, they are usually resistant to standard therapy, which relies on provoking an immune response to the human papilloma virus to eradicate the infection. This is lacking in immunodeficiency.

The infection is overwhelming in nature

Scabies, generalized without the typical reaction, is often found in the immunocompromised. Syphilis can be very florid in the HIV patient.

One should remember that overall immunodeficiency is rare. The majority of patients that have cutaneous infections will have normal immunity.

6.28 Are there any other skin problems seen in patients with HIV infection?

In addition to obvious infections, the patient with HIV can have one or more of several other skin manifestations. In some instances skin disease can be the initial clue that the patient is harbouring HIV.

A few weeks after acquisition of HIV, many patients have a glandular fever-like illness, very often with a pink maculopapular rash. This can be widespread and usually involves the face, palms and soles. It may be months or years after infection before problems relating to immune deficiency occur and one of the most common is severe and often treatment-resistant seborrhoeic dermatitis. Many patients with AIDS have very dry skin and/or generalized pruritus. Itchy papular eruptions, particularly on the face and trunk, are also common in patients with untreated, established HIV, and, especially if sterile pustules are seen, the diagnosis is likely to be eosinophilic folliculitis. Psoriasis can be more florid and atypical in HIV patients.

Although Kaposi's sarcoma is the most well known of the skin cancers associated with HIV, other forms of skin cancer are actually more common (e.g. anogenital squamous carcinoma and lymphomas).

Therapy for HIV is also associated with a number of dermatological problems. Notable is a distinctive lipodystrophy in which there is a loss of fat from the face and extremities, and accumulation centrally. This mainly occurs with the protease inhibitors. Drug eruptions are common and often severe (e.g. Stevens–Johnson syndrome).

 PATIENT QUESTIONS

6.29 Is a cold sore caused by the same virus as herpes?

The other name for a cold sore is herpes simplex. It is, therefore, caused by a herpes virus. Some people use the term 'herpes' for genital herpes which is also caused by the herpes simplex virus. It used to be thought that two types of herpes simplex accounted separately for cold sores and genital herpes – type 1 and type 2 respectively. Nowadays it is less clear cut.

6.30 Can you catch shingles from chickenpox?

Shingles is caused by the chickenpox virus which is another herpes virus. Shingles comes from the reactivation of the virus in someone who has had chickenpox in the past. You cannot catch shingles from chickenpox but someone who has never had chickenpox could catch it from contact with a patch of shingles.

6.31 Is shingles a sign that something is seriously wrong – such as having cancer?

This used to be taught, but without any real evidence. More recently the evidence suggests that there is no connection between shingles and a diagnosis of cancer in those under the age of 65. There was some suggestion that cancer was more likely in women over 65 with shingles but this seemed to be more than a year after the attack of shingles so there may not be any real connection – just a statistical one.

6.32 My son keeps catching impetigo. What can I do to prevent it?

He may be getting recurrent infections from someone in the family who carries the particular bacterium without showing signs of the infection. He could himself carry it in the nostrils. This is why we recommend that swabs are taken from various sites on the body for all close contacts in case some extra treatment is necessary. Your son might also benefit from an antiseptic wash used instead of soap.

6.33 Are warts and verrucas the same thing?

Yes, they are both caused by the same virus. The difference comes from the site of infection – on the soles the pressure drives the affected skin deep instead of allowing it to grow out as in a typical wart.

Fungal infections

7.1   How common is tinea of the scalp?

Tinea capitis mainly occurs in children and adolescents. There is great variation in the epidemiology depending on location. In many British cities with populations of Caribbean or African descent there has been a marked increase in the number of cases seen in recent years, mainly among these populations. The cause is usually *Trichophyton tonsurans*, an anthropophilic fungus. In rural areas and some European cities without significant immigrant populations the fungi causing tinea capitis are more often of animal origin.

7.2   Why does tinea capitis affect children more than adults?

This is probably because of differences in sebum excretion between children and adults and also the more frequent contact that children have with other hair (e.g. in a crowded classroom).

7.3   Does tinea capitis cause hair loss?

Tinea capitis is most easily recognized because it is a cause of hair loss. This occurs because the fungus invades the hair shafts and weakens them. Some species result in the hair breaking off flush with the scalp, producing an appearance of black dots on the hairless skin; others cause the hair to break at a length of a few millimetres. Hair loss also occurs when there is an inflammatory reaction causing pustules and crusting – in its most extreme form, a boggy mass called a kerion.

Hair loss does not always occur in tinea capitis – sometimes there is just patchy scaling. Apart from where a kerion has caused tissue destruction, regrowth is the norm as the hair follicles are not affected. It is useful to be able to reassure worried children and parents that, several months after treatment, their hair will be normal again.

7.4   What is the best treatment for tinea capitis in children?

This is not an easy question. The only effective treatments are the oral antifungals, and you should know which species you are treating, so always send material for culture.

Griseofulvin is the only effective agent licensed for use in children, but is not currently available in liquid form, so tablets have to be crushed. It has to be given for at least 6 weeks, and in higher than normal doses for the increasingly common *Trichophyton tonsurans*. Terbinafine is at least as effective as griseofulvin for most species but is less effective against *Microsporum canis*. It is given for 4 weeks at a dose of 62.5 mg (quarter tablet) for children up to 20 kg body weight, 125 mg (half tablet) for 20–40 kg and 250 mg for 40 kg and above. Fluconazole 0.3 mg/kg/day and itraconazole 3 mg/kg/day are also effective and liquid forms are available but, like terbinafine, these are not licensed for dermatophyte infections in children. They can still be used but parents must be aware that this is in line with 'accepted practice' and not a licensed indication.

Transmission of the causative fungus may be reduced by use of an antifungal shampoo (e.g. one containing 2% ketoconazole or selenium sulphide) but this is not sufficient as treatment.

7.5 What about treating tinea on the rest of the body?

For most localized infections of the skin, topical terbinafine is the most rapidly effective agent. When palms or soles are affected, when hair follicles are involved (e.g. tinea faciei and steroid-treated tinea), and for nail infection, an oral antifungal is indicated. The newer drugs are preferable to griseofulvin, and of these terbinafine has the advantages of fewer drug interactions than itraconazole. There is less published experience with fluconazole. For very inflamed or itchy 'ringworm' on the body a combined preparation containing hydrocortisone and an azole drug such as miconazole can be useful.

7.6 Why don't children seem to get tinea of the nails?

They do, but much less often than is seen in adults. This may be due to a faster growth rate in young nails. When it does occur it is usually when there are adults with tinea pedis and/or nail disease in the family.

7.7 Does tinea unguium always need months of treatment?

Fingernails respond better than toenails – 6 weeks' oral terbinafine (or 2–3 months itraconazole) is usually curative. For toenails, there is a failure rate with all the oral agents, even when they are given for several months and a topical agent such as amorolfine nail lacquer is used as well. Any factor reducing nail growth, such as peripheral vascular disease, will reduce the likelihood of success. For one or perhaps a few affected nails, avulsion or chemical dissolution with 40% urea paste may be a better option than an oral antifungal.

As growth can be very slow, repeated samples should be sent for mycology after 3 months of treatment. The medication may have worked and can be stopped, but the nail itself can take a year to grow back to normal. After severe infections, the nail may never look completely normal so it is very important to avoid unnecessary prolongation of the course of treatment.

By tinea unguium we mean dermatophyte infection; if the culture yields a mould, the above remarks do not apply, so, as for the scalp, you should always send material for mycology.

7.8 What would be the risks of not treating tinea unguium?

Nail infections can be painful. Bacterial infection of the soft tissue (paronychia) can occur secondary to a distorted fungally infected toenail, and particularly in the diabetic this can have serious consequences. Recurrent attacks of cellulitis can result from this secondary bacterial infection. In the immunocompromised, fusarium has been described arising from a nail infection and becoming disseminated.

7.9 Is pityriasis versicolor a fungal infection?

Pityriasis versicolor is a superficial infection caused by Malassezia yeasts; yeasts are fungi so the answer is, yes! It presents as patches of variable pigment, usually on the trunk. It is commonly seen after a holiday as the action of the yeast prevents tanning in the infected skin so paler patches are seen with a fine scale on close examination. If the skin has not been exposed to the sun and remains pale, the affected patches look darker than the surrounding skin – hence the name 'versicolor'.

7.10 How do you treat pityriasis versicolor and how can recurrence be prevented?

Several different topical treatments work well. These include the azole antifungals, terbinafine cream and selenium sulphide. Lotions may be more rapidly effective than creams, so ketoconazole and selenium sulphide shampoos are good choices. They can be applied directly to the skin after a 50% dilution with water, allowed to dry and washed off in the shower. This should be repeated for 3 days in 1 week. If the infection is very widespread, oral itraconazole 200 mg daily for 7 days is usually very effective. Treated areas often remain hypopigmented for months so patients should be advised against unnecessary repeat treatments.

Recurrences are common, so prophylaxis can be achieved with a single dose of itraconazole 400 mg once monthly or with intermittent applications of itraconazole or selenium sulphide shampoo once a month or so.

7.11 Mycology tests sometimes seem to be reported as negative even with clinically obvious fungal infection. Is it useful to send samples?

It is worth sending samples but they need to be taken properly and sent to a laboratory with a specialized mycology department. Fungi can be difficult to culture and good departments have a much lower rate of false negative reporting. When taking a sample from a suspected fungal skin infection it is important to scrape across the edge of the lesion (*Fig. 7.1*). This is where the fungus is most active.

Scraping should be done with a blunt scalpel or similar blade held perpendicularly and the lesions should not have had any recent topical treatments.

Nails can be clipped and have any crumbly material under them scraped out. Clippings and scrapings should be wrapped in black paper before being sent to the laboratory.

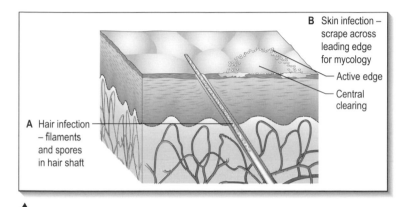

B Skin infection – scrape across leading edge for mycology

Active edge

Central clearing

A Hair infection – filaments and spores in hair shaft

Fig. 7.1 **A** A hair in its follicle showing fungal spores in the hair shaft. **B** Superficial patch of fungal infection of the skin illustrating the scraping technique to obtain samples for mycology.

7.12 What information should be put on the form sent with the sample?

It is very important to include information that might alert the laboratory to the need to look for unusual fungi. As well as mentioning the suspected diagnosis, details of any contact with animals, other cases or recent foreign travel should be included. For nail infections it is useful to note any pre-existing damage to the affected nail as this may make mould infection more likely.

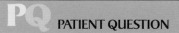

PATIENT QUESTION

7.13 How can I prevent repeated attacks of athlete's foot?

The fungus causing athlete's foot is often caught around swimming pools and in other places where communal changing is the norm so avoidance can help. You need to make sure that each attack is thoroughly treated and that you examine carefully between all the toes for any untreated bits. Nail disease will not be treated by creams and might need a course of tablets.

Shoes can be a source of reinfection as spores can survive in them and get back onto the skin. A dusting with one of the commercial antifungal foot powders can help. The powders are of no use in treating established infection.

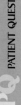

Reactive erythemas and vasculitis

8

8.1 Why are these conditions grouped together?

The conditions grouped as 'reactive erythemas' are urticaria, erythema multiforme and erythema nodosum. In each of these conditions blood vessels are targeted by an inflammatory process and become dilated, resulting in skin lesions that are red and there is usually some degree of swelling of the affected skin. In most vasculitic skin lesions there will be purpura due to the leakage of red blood cells into the tissues in addition to erythema. The term vasculitis means an inflammatory process of the walls of blood vessels and although a pathologist likes to see evidence in a biopsy of destructive changes as well as the presence of inflammation, there is overlap in the appearances and possible underlying causes of the reactive erythemas and the different types of vasculitis.

URTICARIA

8.2 What is urticaria?

The hallmark of urticaria is the weal (wheal, welt or hive). This is an acute, short-lived, localized pink swelling with no surface alteration, due to leakiness of the small blood vessels. The amount of fluid leaked may be so great as to compress nearby vessels, making the centre of the weal paler than the edge.

Urticarial weals rarely last more than 24 hours, fade completely and have no surface alterations; a differential diagnosis should be considered if the lesions last days or weeks (e.g. insect bite), if there is surface alteration – for example, blisters forming might point towards pemphigoid or an eczema – or some lesions become purpuric (consider vasculitis). When the episode of weals lasts less than 6 weeks the urticaria is said to be acute and, if longer than this, it is termed chronic.

If the process occurs in the subcutaneous tissue, the lesions are often less red and less well defined; this is called angioedema. This may occur alone or with typical urticarial weals.

8.3 What are the causes of urticaria?

Urticaria is a result of the release of histamine and other substances from mast cells near small blood vessels, causing them to dilate and become leaky.

When the bout of urticaria is very short (e.g. a few days), a cause is more likely to be apparent than in chronic urticaria. Examples include a recent infectious illness (usually upper respiratory tract infection), a new medication (especially a non-steroidal anti-inflammatory drug, NSAID) and food, with common culprits being shellfish or nuts. When urticaria is due to allergy, the usual mechanism is an interaction between the allergen and IgE antibodies bound to the surface of mast cells. Chronic urticaria includes the physical types, urticaria of unknown cause and urticaria as part of a generalized illness (*Box 8.1*).

Physical urticarias

Physical urticarias are recognized by the trigger: these include dermatographism (caused by friction, e.g. stroking or scratching), delayed deep pressure (e.g. from walking and sitting), cold and solar radiation (the weals have the time course of urticaria – contrast with polymorphic light eruption, Q 5.9). Often included with the physical urticarias is cholinergic urticaria. In this distinctive condition, with tiny weals surrounded by red flares, the immediate cause is a sudden onset of sweating – for example from a rise in environmental temperature, exercise or emotional upset. It can be intensely itchy.

Chronic urticaria not due to a physical stimulus

This type of urticaria is usually of unknown cause, although it can be worsened in some people by ingestion of the food additives benzoates and salicylates. Many foods also contain naturally occurring salicylates which often complicate the picture. The underlying mechanism in at least some patients with chronic urticaria is autoimmune, i.e. there is a circulating IgG antibody directed against either IgE or the IgE receptor bound to mast cells.

Systemic urticaria

Occasionally urticaria is associated with a systemic illness; examples include systemic lupus erythematosus (SLE), the serum sickness reaction and internal parasitic infestation.

BOX 8.1 Types of urticaria

- Ordinary urticaria (idiopathic)
  — acute
  — chronic
- Physical
  — cold, light frictional pressure (dermographism), delayed pressure, solar, heat, vibration
- Cholinergic
- Allergic
- Pharmacological
- Contact urticaria
- Angioedema

Contact urticaria

Contact urticaria is distinguished by the weals occurring only where the skin has been directly exposed to the causative agent. Most examples are due to an IgE-based allergic response. Examples include urticaria when licked by a pet and a localized reaction to latex in rubber gloves.

Angioedema

Angioedema occurs primarily in the subcutaneous tissues. Common sites are around the eyes, mouth, in the genital areas and the loose skin on tops of hands and feet. It may be associated with swelling of the tongue and larynx.

When there is angioedema but no urticaria, it may be necessary to consider hereditary angioedema. In this condition there is a deficiency of the inhibitor of C_1 esterase and C_4 levels are low. As well as angioedema there can be recurrent attacks of abdominal pain and vomiting, often before the skin signs appear, and an autosomal dominant family history.

8.4 Are there useful investigations in the diagnosis of urticaria?

In most cases a careful history is sufficient. A description of the nature and duration of lesions should enable urticaria to be distinguished from other inflammatory processes. The circumstances at the time of the onset may point to an infectious or drug trigger (remember to ask about all non-prescribed medicines), the physical urticarias and some obvious allergic causes.

If allergy is a possibility, and particularly when angioedema has occurred, confirmation of IgE-based reactions may be possible by appropriate skin prick tests or sending serum for radioallergosorbent tests (RASTs) to specific allergens. It can be particularly worth doing tests when the patient has been exposed to several possible allergens, or is uncertain about whether the insect that caused a severe reaction was a wasp or a bee.

For suspected drugs, in general tests are not feasible, with the exception of penicillin, for which a positive test is informative (but a negative result does not exclude penicillin allergy).

For angioedema in the absence of urticaria, C1 esterase inhibitor and C4 should be checked.

In some cases of chronic urticaria there may be a clue from the history or examination for a systemic disease which will suggest worthwhile further investigations. If not, it is reasonable to check a full blood count and differential white cell count, ESR or plasma viscosity, autoimmune screen, hepatitis serology, thyroid tests and a chest radiograph.

8.5   How should urticaria be managed?

It is always worth looking for a cause, or at least categorizing the urticaria (*see Box 8.1*). Where the cause is an allergy, the trigger should be avoided. For physical urticarias and cholinergic urticaria, the triggers should be minimized as best possible. The most appropriate symptomatic treatment is a non-sedative H_1 antihistamine, the easiest for the patient being those with a long duration of action (e.g. fexofenadine, loratadine and cetirizine). If the benefit does not last 24 hours, it may be worth adding a sedative antihistamine such as hydroxyzine at bed time. Sometimes modest additional benefit can be achieved by adding an H_2 antihistamine (e.g. cimetidine), the beta agonist terbutaline or a leukotriene antagonist such as montelukast. In pregnancy, the safest option is one of the old fashioned sedative antihistamines such as chlorpheniramine or diphenhydramine.

Because aspirin and NSAIDs can aggravate as well as cause urticaria, they are probably best avoided in all cases of chronic urticaria.

ERYTHEMA MULTIFORME

8.6   What is erythema multiforme?

The distinguishing features of erythema multiforme are the presence of at least a few target lesions and the typical location of the lesions. The target lesion has a purple or sometimes blistering centre, then a ring of pallor and beyond that an outer ring of erythema. The common sites affected are the hands, feet, elbows and knees. Lesions are often painful rather than itchy, and may last 1–2 weeks.

Skin lesions may be associated with mucosal ulceration, especially the buccal mucosa and lips, conjunctivae, nose and genital area. When this is severe, the term Stevens–Johnson syndrome may be used. This can overlap with toxic epidermal necrolysis, in which large areas of skin become acutely inflamed progressing on to blistering and resulting in the shedding of large areas of epidermis. Epidermal necrolysis is, therefore, a medical emergency.

8.7   What are the causes of erythema multiforme?

Most cases in which a cause is suspected are due to a preceding infection or drug. Infections seen with some frequency include herpes simplex and mycoplasma (in children). Many drugs have been implicated, particularly sulphonamides, antibiotics, anticonvulsants, NSAIDs and allopurinol. Unusual causes include lupus erythematosus, radiotherapy and malignancies. When erythema multiforme is recurrent, the most common cause is recurrent herpes simplex even if not clinically apparent.

In practice, a cause for erythema multiforme is often never found.

8.8 How should erythema multiforme be managed?

Any suspect drug should be stopped, and other causes (e.g. infection) treated if possible. Most cases of erythema multiforme without significant mucosal ulceration will only need symptomatic treatment (e.g. a potent topical steroid). If there is significant involvement of the ocular, oral and/or urogenital mucosa, hospital treatment may well be required. If an episode is recognized sufficiently early, oral corticosteroids may be helpful.

A patient with recurrent or persistent erythema multiforme may require investigation for an underlying cause and, if none is found, a trial of treatment with prophylactic aciclovir should be considered.

ERYTHEMA NODOSUM

8.9 What is erythema nodosum?

Erythema nodosum is distinguished by the outbreak of red nodules, usually tender and typically over the shins, sometimes on the extensor surface of the forearms and occasionally at other sites. There are often some joint symptoms, sometimes a fever and lymphadenopathy. The episode may last as long as a few weeks; as the lesions settle they show the colour changes of an evolving bruise.

8.10 What are the causes of erythema nodosum?

There are many recognized triggers for erythema nodosum, and the likelihood of finding a cause will depend in part on the prevalence of relevant infections. Some of the causes of erythema nodosum are listed in *Box 8.2.*

Appropriate tests are full blood count, differential white cell count, ESR or plasma viscosity, throat swab, ASOT titre, chest radiograph; if there is diarrhoea, stool examination and if there is any likelihood of exposure, skin tests for relevant infectious agents (e.g. tuberculosis, coccidioidomycosis).

It is not uncommon for no cause to be found.

8.11 In erythema nodosum do you treat the rash or the cause?

Whatever the cause, anything but a mild attack will settle more quickly with rest and elevation of the legs (this may mean bed rest), together with a non-steroidal anti-inflammatory analgesic.

If there is an infective cause which will not spontaneously remit, then this should be treated. If sarcoidosis is suspected, further evaluation is needed, and treatment may be necessary (e.g. for iritis). Clearly if an association such as inflammatory bowel disease or a lymphoma is discovered, treatment will be determined by that disease. If the cause may be a drug, this should be discontinued.

BOX 8.2 **Some causes of erythema nodosum**

Infections
- *Streptococcus pyogenes*
- Tuberculosis
- *Lymphogranuloma venereum*
- *Yersinia enterocolitica*
- Salmonella
- Campylobacter
- Mycoplasma
- Coccidioidomycosis, histoplasmosis and blastomycosis

Drugs
- Sulphonamides
- Oral contraceptives

Systemic disease
- Sarcoidosis
- Inflammatory bowel disease (ulcerative colitis or Crohn's)
- Behçet's disease
- Lymphoma, e.g. Hodgkin's disease

VASCULITIS

8.12 What is vasculitis?

Vasculitis means inflammation involving the blood vessel wall. As well as inflammatory cells being present, a biopsy will show evidence of damage – for example, swelling of endothelial cells, obliteration of the lumen, and deposition of fibrin within and beyond the vessel wall. These structural changes are not seen in the 'reactive erythemas' such as urticaria and erythema nodosum.

Vasculitis may be confined to the skin, but the skin lesions may be an important sign of a multisystem disease. As well as non-specific symptoms such as fever, weight loss, muscle and joint aches, vasculitis can affect almost all organs and body systems. Recognition of a specific syndrome is important because there are characteristic patterns of organ involvement (e.g. the respiratory tract and kidneys in Wegener's granulomatosis).

There are many causes of vasculitis, and yet a particular cause can result in a number of different presentations (e.g. streptococcal infection can trigger Henoch–Schönlein purpura or systemic polyarteritis nodosa). Nonetheless even after careful investigation, sometimes no cause is found.

> Not all that looks like vasculitis is vasculitis; it can be mimicked by obstruction of vessels – for example, by septic and cholesterol emboli, and cryoglobulins.

8.13 Why does vasculitis present in different ways?

There is a wide range of clinical appearances in the skin which can all have vasculitis as their underlying mechanism. These include lesions which resemble urticaria but last longer and resolve with the colour change of a fading bruise; purpuric papules, nodules and plaques; and deeper nodules with overlying normal skin. Secondary events due to ischaemia or infarction of overlying skin include blisters, ulceration, eschar formation and even gangrene. Sometimes the skin shows subtle changes which may imply vasculitis such as livedo reticularis, even though this is not necessarily directly due to the vasculitis itself.

These differences are usually explained by one or more of:

■ the size and type of vessel affected, i.e. venule, vein, arteriole or artery
■ the degree of vascular obliteration
■ how much inflammation occurs
■ the chronicity of the process
■ the cause.

8.14 What are the causes of vasculitis?

Triggers for vasculitis include:

■ infections, e.g. *Streptococcus pyogenes*, subacute bacterial endocarditis, hepatitis B and C, tuberculosis
■ drugs – prescribed, over-the-counter and illicit
■ malignancies, especially haematological
■ connective tissue disease, e.g. SLE, rheumatoid
■ other systemic disease.

Mechanisms include:

■ immune complexes lodging in vessel walls
■ antineutrophil cytoplasmic antibodies (ANCA)
■ antiphospholipid antibodies.

8.15 What happens when vasculitis affects small vessels?

The small vessels involved are typically the venules into which the capillaries drain. They are located in the superficial dermis. Inflammation is usually due to neutrophils, sometimes eosinophils, or both. In a few diseases (e.g. lupus erythematosus) lymphocytes are usually responsible. If the inflammation does not result in occlusion of the vessel, the lesions are likely to resemble urticaria but will last longer – and because there has been damage there will be some leakage of red blood cells. Even if this does not produce purpura, when the lesions resolve there will be some brown discolouration from haemosiderin in the tissue which may take 1–2 weeks to fade. More severe inflammation will result in purpuric papules and plaques, which can be painful. These lesions can blister, and even ulcerate before healing. The most common site is the lower limbs.

Small vessel vasculitis (SVV) may affect just the skin, but can be the skin manifestation of a systemic vasculitis such as Henoch–Schönlein purpura. SVV can also occur in diseases characterized by vasculitis of arteries such as systemic polyarteritis nodosa and Churg–Strauss syndrome, and in autoimmune diseases (mainly SLE and rheumatoid disease).

8.16 How different is large vessel vasculitis?

There are a few clues that larger vessels might be affected. These include:

- subcutaneous nodules
- gangrene in the territory of an affected artery, e.g. a finger or toe
- livedo reticularis (a net-like purplish discolouration), especially when the net is incomplete or broken.

Vasculitis of larger vessels includes systemic polyarteritis nodosa (PAN), Wegener's granulomatosis, Churg–Strauss syndrome, temporal arteritis and Takayasu's arteritis. Sometimes evidence for one of these diseases will come from a skin biopsy which includes the diagnostic histopathology. Usually there is clinical evidence of internal organ involvement such as renal disease (PAN or Wegener's), or asthma (Churg–Strauss).

It should be noted that the circumstances in which large vessel vasculitis occurs (e.g. PAN and Wegener's) are often accompanied by small vessel vasculitis as well.

8.17 How should vasculitis be managed?

Vasculitis presenting in the skin can look the same whether it is an isolated event or part of a systemic process. There might be a cause and it might be treatable.

The approach to the patient should be to use clinical clues and appropriate investigations to evaluate whether the patient is ill and what other organs might be affected, and to search for a cause. If a drug is suspected it should be withdrawn. Any likely infection should be treated. If another organ system is affected (e.g. the kidneys), this may well determine the decision as to whether to treat, and with what. More than with most skin presentations, a full clinical history and examination (including blood pressure) are essential.

A biopsy of a fresh skin lesion for histology will at least support the diagnosis of vasculitis; if a sample can be submitted for frozen section or in Michel's medium for direct immunofluorescence, this can be useful. If the lesions are deep, a formal elliptical biopsy should be taken.

In all cases it is generally wise to check the urine for red cells, white cells, casts and protein, a full blood count and differential white cell count, and ESR or plasma viscosity, and appropriate tests for any suspected infection on the basis of symptoms and signs. If no cause is found, further tests that may be useful include autoantibodies (ANA, ENA screen, dsDNA and rheumatoid factor), complement C3 and C4, ANCA, antiphospholipid antibodies, immunoglobulins and electrophoretic strip, cryoglobulins, hepatitis B and C serology, streptococcal antibodies and a chest radiograph.

If a bout of vasculitis does not settle spontaneously, it may be prudent to repeat the investigations for a possible cause or internal organ involvement, particularly if there are systemic features such as fever or weight loss.

Cases where significant organ involvement is suspected should be referred to secondary care. Mild cases of purely cutaneous vasculitis with mainly urticarial lesions will usually settle spontaneously. An oral antihistamine may be of help. For more severe cases, systemic corticosteroids may be necessary, but should only be used short term.

 PATIENT QUESTIONS

8.18   My father has a brown speckled rash on his lower legs which is just unsightly. He is well and it doesn't itch – is it serious?

Your father sounds as though he has a pigmented purpuric dermatosis. This descriptive term gives a clue that the cause is unknown. It usually starts on the feet and gradually moves further up the legs. It seems that the blood vessels just leak a little blood without any significant inflammation or vasculitis. The leaked blood gives rise to a bruise – purpura – and the pigmentation is from the deposition of haemosiderin (a blood pigment) in the skin. There is no treatment but your father should avoid soap and use a moisturizer to keep his skin in as good condition as possible.

8.19   My doctor has told me that I can take up to two of my antihistamines (cetirizine) a day to try to control my severe urticaria. The leaflet with the pills only talks about taking one a day – is this safe?

There are many occasions in medicine when drugs are used outwith the terms of their original licence. Cetirizine is one which can be safely used at higher doses and this knowledge has been acquired through experience of treating patients, like you, with difficult urticaria. No-one else reading this should start to take higher doses without discussing it with their doctor.

8.20   I seem to react to aspirin as a cause of my urticaria – what foods should I avoid?

Many different foods contain 'salicylates' which are similar to aspirin and the list, unfortunately, is long. A wide range of citrus and other fruits, both fresh and when dried, should be avoided. Other 'healthy' food such as vegetables can also be a problem, especially beetroot, cauliflower, cabbage, cucumber, French beans, peas, potatoes, peppers, sweetcorn and tomatoes. Beer, wine and some spirits should also be avoided as should pickles and vinegar. It might be easier to look at a list of foods you can eat! Meat, fish, cheese, eggs, milk, bread, rice, pasta, tea and coffee are all safe. You would be wise to consult a dietitian for a full list and advice as to how to maintain a healthy diet for the 6-week period that is necessary to see if your skin improves.

Blistering diseases

9.1 What is a blister?

A blister is a collection of fluid within the skin. The usual site is either within the epidermis or between the epidermis and dermis (*Fig. 9.1*). Sometimes patients (and even doctors) use the term blister for a lesion which is something different (e.g. an urticarial weal). Proof of this being a blister will come if free fluid is released, either spontaneously or after puncture.

9.2 Is there a simple way of classifying blistering diseases?

The simplest approach is by the location within the skin where the blister originates (*Box 9.1*). The deeper the split, the more likely the blister will remain intact and tense.

9.3 What are the most important causes of blisters?

There are many different causes of blisters which are probably best grouped as below.

- Acute eczema: atopic, contact, pompholyx, etc.
- Bacteria: bullous impetigo
- Viruses: herpes simplex and varicella zoster
- Drugs: erythema multiforme/toxic epidermal necrolysis, bullous drug eruption including fixed drug eruption
- Autoimmune: pemphigus, pemphigoid, dermatitis herpetiformis, linear IgA disease, bullous lupus erythematosus
- Genetic: epidermolysis bullosa
- Miscellaneous: heat and cold injury, arthropod bite.

PEMPHIGUS

9.4 What is pemphigus?

Pemphigus vulgaris and pemphigus foliaceous are the two more common members of a family of autoimmune blistering diseases in which there are autoantibodies directed against desmogleins, one of the components of the

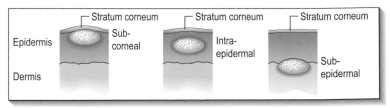

▲

Fig. 9.1 Different levels of blister formation.

BOX 9.1 Blistering diseases – a classification

Subcorneal
- Bullous impetigo
- Staphylococcal scalded skin syndrome
- Pemphigus foliaceous

Intraepidermal
- Acute eczema
- Herpes simplex, zoster and chicken pox
- Pemphigus vulgaris
- Epidermolysis bullosa simplex

Subepidermal
- Bullous pemphigoid
- Dermatitis herpetiformis
- Bullous erythema multiforme
- Toxic epidermal necrolysis
- Bullous insect bite
- Bullous drug eruption
- Porphyria
- Dystrophic epidermolysis bullosa

cell adhesion structure called the desmosome. The antibodies cause cell separation, which then leads to blister formation, often with keratinocytes floating in the fluid (acantholysis).

9.5   How does pemphigus present?

In pemphigus vulgaris the split occurs such that the basal layer of the epidermis forms the floor of the blister. The mouth and sometimes other mucosae are often involved early in the disease, sometimes before the skin is affected. The blisters are typically flaccid and break easily, leaving painful erosions which can become infected. The trunk, flexures and scalp are often involved. Typically, the patient is middle aged. The Nikolsky sign is often positive, i.e. sliding pressure on normal skin will produce separation of the epidermis.

In pemphigus foliaceous a different desmoglein is attacked by the autoimmune process. In contrast to pemphigus vulgaris, the mucosal surfaces are not involved and the split within the epidermis is under the horny layer; fragile blisters may occur but more commonly there are crusts and weeping on an inflamed background. Pemphigus foliaceous usually begins on the trunk and can become widespread.

9.6   How should pemphigus be managed?

Untreated, pemphigus vulgaris can be fatal but, as some of its treatments have potentially severe side effects, it is very important to make a correct diagnosis.

Diagnosis is best made by taking a biopsy of a small fresh lesion for histology, dividing off the skin adjacent to the blister and sending this (fresh, frozen or in Michel's medium) for direct immunofluorescence. The autoantibodies can usually be detected in serum either by indirect immunofluorescence, or better (but less widely available) by ELISA.

In pemphigus vulgaris initial treatment is with high doses of oral corticosteroid to bring the disease under control; for resistant cases pulsed intravenous methylprednisolone and/or cyclophosphamide are sometimes used. For maintenance and steroid sparing, immunosuppressants such as azathioprine are used.

Pemphigus foliaceous is often controlled with lower doses of prednisolone, and potent topical corticosteroids have a role. As with pemphigus vulgaris, a steroid-sparing agent is often required.

In pemphigus the antibody titre is useful in monitoring disease activity, a rise sometimes preceding a worsening of the disease.

PEMPHIGOID

9.7 Is pemphigoid another type of pemphigus?

The pemphigoid family is a different group of autoimmune blistering diseases in which the blister forms with the entire epidermis as the roof. The characteristic autoantibodies react with molecules which are partly or wholly within the basement membrane zone, a complex layer lying between the basal keratinocytes of the epidermis and the papillary dermis. The autoimmune reaction involves immunoglobulin and complement C3 – the latter often being the most easily demonstrated immune reactant – and various inflammatory cells. Some patients have basement membrane-localizing antibodies detectable in serum, usually by indirect immunofluorescence. As with pemphigus, the diagnosis is usually made by both histology and direct immunofluorescence of perilesional skin.

9.8 Are there different types of pemphigoid?

By both clinical and immunopathological criteria there are different types of pemphigoid. The common denominator is confirming the diagnosis by performing direct immunofluorescence on perilesional skin and finding complement C3 and sometimes IgG in the basement membrane zone.

Bullous pemphigoid

This is the commonest autoimmune bullous disease. It mainly occurs in the elderly. There is usually an itchy erythematous eruption before blisters appear. These are tense, sometimes haemorrhagic and can become large. Bullous pemphigoid can be localized (e.g. to one leg) or widespread. The mucous membranes are seldom involved.

Cicatricial (mucous membrane) pemphigoid
Blisters can occur but are uncommon in this variant. The main problem is painful erosions of the oral, conjunctival and genital mucosal surfaces. The condition progresses to scarring, and blindness is a possible outcome.

Pemphigoid gestationis
Once called herpes gestationis, this rare inflammatory and subepidermal blistering disease occurs mainly during pregnancy (the other association is with trophoblastic tumours). Remission usually occurs after the baby is born.

9.9 How should pemphigoid be managed?

When bullous pemphigoid is localized and stable it may respond to a potent or super-potent topical corticosteroid. The first line of treatment for generalized bullous pemphigoid will usually be prednisolone, initially in a dose of up to 60 mg/day depending on severity and early response. If the disease relapses when this is withdrawn, a steroid-sparing agent will be required – often azathioprine.

DERMATITIS HERPETIFORMIS

9.10 What is dermatitis herpetiformis?

This is an intensely itchy papular and vesicular disease. The use of the word 'herpetiformis' suggests a tendency for lesions to be grouped together in the areas of commonest presentation, i.e. the elbows, knees, buttocks, shoulders and in the scalp. It does not indicate any association with herpes virus infections.

9.11 Can blisters always be seen in dermatitis herpetiformis?

No. the condition is so itchy that scratching has usually destroyed the roof of the vesicles so that the presentation is one of multiple small erosions.

9.12 Is dermatitis herpetiformis caused by gluten sensitivity?

Dermatitis herpetiformis is a manifestation of gluten sensitivity but most patients do not have clinically apparent small bowel disease, i.e. coeliac disease. If the small bowel is biopsied, there are often some subtle and patchy changes seen on histology.

9.13 How can a suspected diagnosis be confirmed?

A biopsy should be taken from normal skin as this will show the presence of autoantibodies to, for example, endomysium. The most specific diagnostic finding is the presence of IgA in a granular pattern in the dermal papillae.

9.14 Is dermatitis herpetiformis associated with any other diseases?

As mentioned above (*see Q 9.12*), the small bowel can be affected with malabsorption and symptomatic bowel upset. In the long term there is a risk of small bowel lymphoma. Other autoimmune problems can occur, of which hypothyroidism is the most common, occurring in 14% of patients.

9.15 How should dermatitis herpetiformis be managed?

Treatment involves strict adherence to a gluten-free diet but this takes a long time to be effective. In the interim, drug therapy – usually with dapsone – works well.

LINEAR IGA DISEASE

9.16 What is linear IgA disease?

It is rare but is a unique example of a disease being named after an immunopathological finding – the presence of a linear deposition of IgA and complement C3 at the basement membrane zone. It is clinically similar to dermatitis herpetiformis with intense itching and burning, although blisters can be bigger. There is no associated small bowel disease or gluten sensitivity.

9.17 Does linear IgA disease affect all ages?

Yes, but it presents differently in children and in adults. The childhood form has a predilection for the genito-crural skin and the blisters spread centrifugally to resemble 'strings of pearls' which is taken as a diagnostic sign. In adults there are urticarial plaques and tense blisters which can look more like pemphigoid.

9.18 How should linear IgA disease be managed?

Linear IgA disease responds well to dapsone.

Leg ulcers

10

10.1 What are the essential questions to ask when assessing a patient with a leg ulcer?

Not only are there many possible causes for leg ulceration, but in a particular patient there may be more than one cause. For example, quite commonly at least some degree of arterial impairment is found in patients with venous leg ulcers. In most cases a thorough history and clinical examination will point towards the most likely diagnosis (or diagnoses). At least 80% of leg ulcers are wholly or partly due to increased pressure in the leg veins (*Fig. 10.1*). In addition to causes, it is important to find out about health factors which might contribute to the process or interfere with healing – for example, arterial disease, anaemia, diabetes mellitus, heart failure, cigarette smoking, etc.

10.2 What are the characteristic features of a venous ulcer?

There is often a history of deep vein thrombosis and symptoms and signs of venous hypertension. Patients may complain of a heaviness in the legs and there may be pitting oedema. Other clues are:

- a red, or sometimes bluish tinge to the skin
- brown staining of the skin around the ulcer from haemosiderin deposition after extravasation of red blood cells
- atrophie blanche – patches of white scarring with dilated red capillaries
- lipodermatosclerosis – deep-seated induration from fibrosis and oedema, sometimes with overlying erythema
- dilated subcutaneous veins which can be felt with the patient standing up.

The ulcer itself is often near the medial malleolus, large and quite shallow, with a red base made up of granulation tissue. Healing may be taking place with blurring of the margins from re-epithelialization and small grey 'islands' of new epithelial tissue on the base of the ulcer.

10.3 How do arterial ulcers differ?

There is often a history of claudication or other consequences of arterial disease. The skin will be pale and hairless with poor capillary return and absent or diminished peripheral pulses. The ulcers have a much more 'punched-out' appearance with sharply defined edges. They are deeper with little or no granulation tissue. Common sites are the toes, heels and dorsum

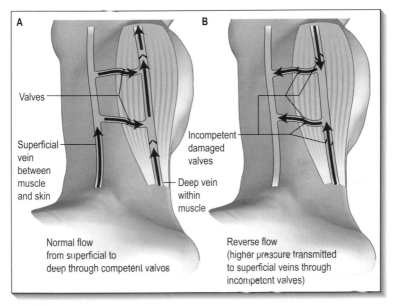

▲

Fig. 10.1 Diagrammatic representation of lower leg illustrating **(A)** normal and **(B)** reverse venous flow.

of the foot but they can also occur on the calves and shins. Doppler testing confirms reduced arterial flow.

10.4 What does a vasculitic ulcer look like?

Like the arterial type, it may well be 'punched out' and deep with sharp edges. The history is more important than the appearance as it will have started with a painful nodule or purpuric plaque. There may be an underlying connective tissue disease such as rheumatoid arthritis, and papules, nodules and purpura may be found on further examination of the patient.

10.5 Can pyoderma gangrenosum present with ulceration?

Yes, and it can look either superficial or deep and destructive. It will probably have started with a tender papule or 'boil' which then broke down. There may be an associated enteropathy, arthritis or haematological disorder (usually leukaemia). The surrounding skin may be blue, overhang the edges of the ulcer and can be blistered or pustular (*see* Q 15.8).

10.6 How would you recognize a malignant ulcer?

The only reliable test is a biopsy but suspicion should be raised if ulceration has occurred in a preceding nodule or plaque. A squamous cell carcinoma may begin in a preceding actinic keratosis or Bowen's disease or complicate a longstanding ulcer. In the latter case, any non-healing ulcer that has been properly assessed and managed should raise the possibility of malignant change. The edge of the ulcer may be heaped up or indurated and the non-ulcerated parts of the lesion may be typical for the type of tumour (e.g. pigmentation in the case of a malignant melanoma).

10.7 Can infection cause ulceration?

This is now rare unless an infection has been acquired in the tropics or the patient is immunosuppressed. Common culprits would be tuberculosis, leprosy or a deep-seated fungal infection such as sporotrichosis. The ulcer will be non-specific with a history of a preceding nodule, plaque or deep-seated pustule.

10.8 Are there any other causes of leg ulceration that should be considered?

It is worth thinking about neuropathy – from diabetes, leprosy or syringomyelia – where ulcers are at site of pressure and have a punched-out appearance with a hyperkeratotic edge. Blood abnormalities such as haemolytic anaemia and polycythaemia can give rise to non-specific, indolent ulcers, and trauma should not be forgotten, especially from repeated pressure around the malleoli.

10.9 Which baseline investigations should be undertaken?

This will depend on the likely aetiology. Specific tests may be required for suspected underlying disease in the case of vasculitic or neuropathic ulcers and in pyoderma gangrenosum but the majority of leg ulcers are venous. In these cases a search for underlying problems or complicating factors such as peripheral vascular disease, obesity, heart failure or arthritis is worthwhile. The urine or blood should be tested for sugar and a full blood count will detect anaemia – a cause of delayed healing – or other, more serious, haematological disorders. A bacterial swab may be taken but all ulcers are infected with bacteria that are clinically unimportant, so this should be restricted to confirming the cause in the presence of obvious clinical signs of infection in the ulcer or surrounding skin. Doppler ultrasound is useful and necessary to exclude arterial problems, especially before compression bandaging (*see Q 10.15*) is used.

10.10 When should a biopsy be done?

When the diagnostic possibilities include malignancy, unusual deep infection or some cases of vasculitis, a biopsy can be the most informative investigation. Biopsies from lower legs, especially those with oedema and poor circulation, may well heal poorly, so there must be good reason to take one.

10.11 What are the basic rules for treating venous ulcers?

The first thing is to establish that it is a venous ulcer without a significant amount of arterial damage. Evaluate the arterial inflow by Doppler ultrasound: if impaired refer for a vascular surgical opinion; if normal proceed onto compression bandaging – either single or multilayer – with a suitable dressing to keep the ulcer surface moist (*Fig. 10.2*). Each review should involve measuring the healing progress by tracing the outline of the ulcer on a transparent sheet to compare it with the previous week. Whenever the dressings are changed, the site should be carefully examined to recognize and treat significant infection (i.e. cellulitis). Allergic response to dressings or creams should be checked for and avoided by minimizing the use of chemicals (e.g. antiseptics which might sensitize or irritate).

10.12 How do you decide between the different types of dressing?

There are a multitude of different dressings out there and local clinicians may have decided on a formulary to help with stock ordering,

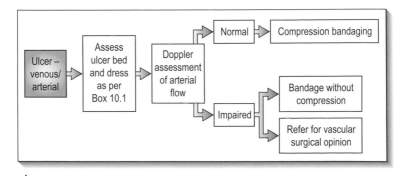

▲
Fig. 10.2 Schematic of treatment for a venous ulcer.

standardization of treatment and budget control. The basic decisions are taken on the basis of the nature of the ulcer bed as shown in *Box 10.1*.

10.13 Are there any other useful topical treatments?

Good fragrance-free emollients in the form of soap substitutes and moisturising creams used around the ulcer will improve the quality and comfort of the surrounding skin. There are a number of additional treatments and additives used on and around ulcers, notably antibiotics, antiseptics and desloughing agents. There is little good evidence to support the use of these, and both allergic and irritant contact dermatitis can occur.

10.14 Are there any systemic treatments that can help healing?

Any underlying diseases should have optimal treatment. There may be some value in taking low-dose aspirin (if tolerated) to improve blood flow in the capillaries around the ulcer. Zinc sulphate and vitamin C are thought, by some, to promote the healing process. Analgesics may be needed as ulcers can be painful and many patients find the compression bandages intolerable. If higher dose aspirin or a non-steroidal anti-inflammatory drug cannot be tolerated, paracetamol can be used. Low-dose amitriptyline can be a useful adjunct to pain relief. Diuretics will be used for heart failure but are of little value for the mechanical oedema associated with venous disease – this is much better treated by compression bandaging (*see Q 10.15*), elevation at rest and exercise.

10.15 What are the principles of compression bandaging?

The purposes of compression bandaging are to reduce oedema, aid venous return and retain dressings.

The leg should be assessed for adequacy of arterial supply, usually by using a hand-held Doppler ultrasound device. The ratio of inflow pressure in the ankle:arm (brachial) is known as the ABPI. Compression bandaging is generally safe if the ABPI is 0.8–1.0.

BOX 10.1 Ulcer bed dressings	
Ulcer bed	**Type of dressing**
Dry, necrotic, black	Hydrocolloid, hydrogel
Yellow, sloughy, moist	Some foam dressings, alginates
Yellow, sloughy, dry	Hydrogel, hydrocolloid
Clean, mildly exuding	Knitted viscose, paraffin tulle, alginates
Malodorous	Dressings with activated charcoal and/or silver
Overgranulating (e.g. after a hydrocolloid)	Foam

The type of bandage is probably less important than the skill and familiarity of the nurse with the product used. When a single stretch bandage is used, the compression is usually not sustained for more than a few days. Multilayer bandages can provide compression which will be sustained for 7 days; if the treatment is well tolerated and exudate does not strike through, this approach can be the most convenient and cost effective.

The bandaging should be applied from the base of the toes to below the knee. If the tension applied is kept constant, the pressure generated beneath the bandage will be graduated – i.e. maximal at the ankle and progressively decreasing proximally. This is because pressure is inversely related to the radius of the leg (a reflection of Laplace's law).

Vulnerable sites beneath the bandaging, such as the malleoli and the skin over the tibia in a thin person, should be protected – for example, by foam or felt pads, and, in the four-layer bandage system, by a generous application of the wool layer.

10.16 When and how should a non-healing ulcer be reassessed?

An uncomplicated venous ulcer should heal if there is adequate compression bandaging, elevation of the leg when the patient is resting, exercising to stimulate venous return through the muscle pump and there are no significant co-morbidities. Such an ulcer is likely to be dressed weekly, and records should be kept of the size, often best done by taking a tracing onto transparent material placed over a layer of cling film on the ulcer, together with the nature of the ulcer surface.

Failure to heal can be due to many factors – for example, infection, eczema, oedema, wrong diagnosis, poor arterial supply, development of squamous cell carcinoma (Marjolin's ulcer), general medical problems (especially anaemia), etc.

If an ulcer is deteriorating or not improving, re-evaluate the ABPI; if there is pus and/or cellulitis, swab and consider an oral antibiotic; if there is increased pain or fever, again consider soft tissue infection. Also consider referral to secondary care if there is concern about the diagnosis, possible malignancy, and in some cases of dermatitis.

10.17 Once the ulcer has healed, what can be done to prevent recurrence?

The most important intervention for the patient with a healed ulcer is provision of graduated support hosiery ever thereafter. These are prescribable. There are three classes of compression (British system): Class 1 is too light to be of much value; Class 2 is suitable for most patients who have a healed venous ulcer; Class 3 is very effective but the stockings are often difficult to put on. The stockings can be thigh length, but most patients get on better with below-knee. Some patients may need a device to help them put the stockings on (e.g. Acti-Glide). Support hosiery should be supplemented with elevation of the legs when resting, exercise and encouragement to lose weight if obese.

PATIENT QUESTIONS

10.18 I have heard that maggots are used to treat ulcers – is that true?

Yes, they are used to treat ulcers. It may sound gruesome but they can play a useful role in cleaning up a lot of dead or damaged tissue over the ulcer surface that will interfere with the healing process. The maggots are specially produced so are quite safe and are kept on the wound under a bandage to clean it up.

10.19 I can't stand compression bandages as they are too painful. What can I do?

This is a common complaint as the pressure needed to achieve healing is quite high. Skilled nurses will apply the bandages correctly to minimize pain and discomfort but it is worth persevering for as long as you can as the pain usually settles once the swelling in the leg goes down. You can ask your doctor for tablets to help – ibuprofen can be a useful painkiller and a small dose of amitriptyline at night might be given if it suited you otherwise.

10.20 What can I do to stop an ulcer coming back?

It is very important to prevent the conditions that caused the ulcer in the first place. If your ulcer is anything other than a venous one, your doctor will be arranging specific treatment; however, with venous ulcers you need to counteract the effect of the damaged veins. The best way to do this is by wearing support hosiery. You should also keep the skin on your legs as healthy as possible with emollients and avoid trauma such as a graze or bad bruise which might lead to the development of an ulcer.

Benign lumps and bumps

11

11.1 What is a naevus?

As words go, for precision this is not one of dermatology's best. The origins of the word naevus lie in Sanskrit and Latin, and refer to birth. In this broad sense are included anomalies presenting at birth, or thought to begin during gestation. Thus, a port-wine stain (a vascular malformation), a haemangioma of infancy (a self-limiting benign tumour) and a shagreen patch (a collagenous hamartoma that is a marker of tuberous sclerosis) are all naevi. Melanocytic naevi may be congenital, but are far commoner as a postnatal event. These acquired melanocytic naevi, usually called moles by the lay public (and often by physicians), are probably what is implied if the word naevus is used without any qualifying adjective.

11.2 Do benign moles change over time?

Yes, so it is not true that any change in a mole is an indication of malignant change.

A mole typically begins as a proliferation of melanocytes at the dermo-epidermal junction. At this stage the clinical presentation is a circumscribed flat brown patch and is termed a junctional naevus. This may progress to a papule or nodule by further proliferation of the melanocytes which move into the dermis; the lesion is now termed a compound naevus. The presence of proliferating melanocytes at the dermo-epidermal junction eventually ceases and the mole is then an intradermal naevus (*Fig. 11.1*). At this stage of its 'life' the mole has often lost its pigment and is flesh-coloured.

Most moles (melanocytic naevi) appear during childhood and adolescence, and evolve during early and mid adulthood. It is relatively uncommon for a new mole to arise from the fifth decade onwards.

11.3 Are some moles more dangerous than others?

Very few moles will ever become malignant melanomas.

Atypical or dysplastic moles

Moles that are somewhat irregular in outline and colour, and have some redness, are termed 'atypical' and often have a histological appearance termed 'dysplastic'. When such a mole is seen to be increasing in size it can be indistinguishable from a melanoma. These moles may themselves have an increased risk of becoming malignant. A person with many atypical moles has an increased risk for melanoma. If there are close family members with multiple atypical moles and there is a familial occurrence of melanoma, then the presence of such moles signifies a very high risk for the

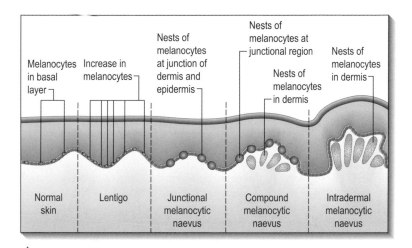

▲

Fig. 11.1 Diagrammatic representation of lesions derived from melanocytes. (Reproduced with kind permission from Kneebone R, Schofield J 1998 Minor surgery and skin lesions: diagnosis and management on CD-ROM. Primal Pictures, London.)

individual. The term familial melanoma syndrome is applied to this population.

Giant congenital melanocytic naevus
If a mole present at birth is predicted to become 20 mm or more when the infant is fully grown, there is a lifetime risk of around 5% for melanoma.

11.4 What causes seborrhoeic warts?

In most cases the cause is unknown. In some families, there is an autosomal dominant tendency to develop numerous seborrhoeic warts. Very rarely, a sudden outbreak of large numbers of seborrhoeic warts is triggered by an internal malignancy (the sign of Leser–Trélat).

Sunlight may play a role in some individuals, especially when the lesions are predominantly on sun-exposed sites.

11.5 How can you tell a seborrhoeic wart from a mole?

A typical seborrhoeic wart looks as though it has been stuck on the skin, i.e. it has no depth. It has a warty appearance and texture, often a colour that is at least partly grey and close inspection (you may need a magnifying glass for this) often reveals tiny rounded yellowish structures (actually minute keratin cysts) and horny plugs within it. If you gently bend up a seborrhoeic wart between finger and thumb you may see clefts running through it. Moles can have a warty surface, but can be seen to occupy some depth in the skin and are a more pure brown in colour.

11.6 Do seborrhoeic warts need treatment?

On medical grounds alone, the answer is, no. Seborrhoeic warts are benign. They can, however, mimic malignant melanoma and epithelial cancers. They can be itchy, catch on clothing, and be unsightly. Removal may therefore be needed for diagnosis or because of nuisance value.

11.7 What is the best treatment for seborrhoeic warts?

For a histological diagnosis, shave biopsy or curettage will provide an adequate sample. Various destructive methods are suitable – curettage, liquid nitrogen cryotherapy or chemical destruction with trichloroacetic acid. Care should be taken not to produce scarring.

11.8 What is a dermatofibroma?

Dermatofibroma, also known as fibrous histiocytoma, is a benign dermal tumour. It is most commonly found on the limbs, has a firm to hard consistency and feels like a pebble tethered to the epidermis when picked up between finger and thumb.

Dermatofibromas can vary widely in colour. They can be painful, and even when asymptomatic may be tender to palpation. As they arise from the dermis, full excision is necessary if removal is required; a simple shave excision would only remove the top layer and allow for regrowth.

11.9 Are sebaceous cysts and epidermoid cysts the same?

No. The entity often referred to as a sebaceous cyst has a wall resembling epidermis and the contents are the same as produced by epidermis, i.e. solid keratinous material. The correct term for this is epidermoid cyst, not sebaceous cyst.

The true sebaceous cyst has lobules of sebaceous gland connected to it and oily contents. Multiple such cysts occur predominantly on the trunk in the inherited condition steatocystoma multiplex.

11.10 Do lipomas cause pain?

Occasionally, but most lipomas do not cause symptoms. Pressure over a lipoma can be painful, as can fat necrosis within one.

Angiolipoma is a histological variant, and represents about 10% of lipomatous lesions excised. Angiolipomas are often painful.

11.11 What is a pyogenic granuloma?

A pyogenic granuloma is a common benign vascular tumour with a completely misleading name. It is not infectious, i.e. not pyogenic, nor is it granulomatous. Pyogenic granulomas particularly occur in young people, sometimes after an injury. They grow quite quickly, are bright red, and are often pedunculated with a surrounding collarette of thickened horny layer. They can bleed profusely when traumatized and acquire a crusted surface.

An important differential diagnosis is amelanotic malignant melanoma.

11.12 How should a pyogenic granuloma be treated?

Treatment is appropriate for lesions where the diagnosis is uncertain, bleeding is a problem, and there is discomfort or disfigurement.

If feasible, excise a pyogenic granuloma and send it for histology. Recurrence is more likely after other types of removal such as curettage.

11.13 What is the difference between a hypertrophic scar and a keloid?

Hypertrophic scar and keloid are both an overgrowth of fibrous tissue following injury, are raised, and early on are redder than the skin nearby. Both can itch and be tender.

A hypertrophic scar remains confined to the borders of the initial injury and will regress at least to some extent after 1–2 years; keloids (from the Greek 'crab claw') extend into tissue beyond the injury and do not regress. Often hypertrophic scar and keloid can only be distinguished with hindsight.

11.14 Can keloids/hypertrophic scars be easily treated?

No single treatment is suitable for all keloids/hypertrophic scars.

Perhaps the easiest treatment is application of silicone – as a gel sheet or fine film of gel from a tube – kept in place all the time except when washing, for up to 1 year. Devices and garments which apply pressure can be successful for some parts of the body. Haelan tape and intralesional corticosteroid injections may be helpful but can produce atrophy, hypopigmentation and telangiectasia. Other treatments used include radiotherapy, interferons and some types of laser (*see* Q 3.21). In experienced hands surgery combined with another modality (e.g. injected steroid or radiotherapy) might be appropriate.

11.15 Is a keratoacanthoma benign or malignant?

A typical keratoacanthoma is a self-limited, well-circumscribed symmetrical tumour with a central keratin-filled crater which grows rapidly but then involutes. Although a typical keratoacanthoma has benign behaviour, some lesions begin like a keratoacanthoma but subsequently behave as squamous carcinoma.

It is probably best to regard keratoacanthoma as a special type of squamous cell carcinoma which has a built-in self-destruct mechanism. Since this cannot be deduced for certain, many prefer to regard even a typical keratoacanthoma as a potential squamous cell carcinoma and treat it as such, usually by excision.

The cosmetic end result of leaving a keratoacanthoma to resolve spontaneously is often an unsightly scar, so it is generally preferable to remove even a typical keratoacanthoma (and of course send for histology) and plan the repair to minimize the resultant scar.

 PATIENT QUESTION

11.16 How would I know if a mole was really a skin cancer?

It is very rare to see new moles appearing after the age of 30 so you should report new ones to your doctor. Moles tend to be regular in colour with a well-defined border and change slowly, if they change at all, so any rapid growth, alteration of colour or change of shape should be looked for. Bleeding without having damaged the mole could be a bad sign but itching is not very important on its own. A good rule of thumb is that if you are not sure, seek advice.

Skin cancer

12.1 What are the different types of skin cancer?

Cancers can probably arise from any of the cell types found in the skin. In addition to these, leukaemia and lymphoma can involve the skin and metastases from internal organs occasionally present cutaneously.

The commonest skin cancers come from the epidermal lineage and are referred to as basal cell and squamous cell carcinomas. Together, these two are grouped and labelled as 'non-melanoma skin cancer'. This is partly because they are not as serious as malignant melanomas which arise from melanocytes.

Other primary skin cancers include Merkel cell tumours, cancers of the skin appendage cells (e.g. sebaceous carcinoma) and various sarcomas. Kaposi's sarcoma, now known to be caused by human herpes virus 8, is a malignancy of blood and lymphatic endothelial cells and is often multifocal in the skin.

12.2 How common is skin cancer?

It depends on the population being studied and the cumulative exposure to the main environmental causes. In Wales in the late 1990s, the incidence of non-melanoma skin cancer was 250 per 100 000. Of these, about one-sixth were squamous cell carcinomas with the remainder being basal cell carcinomas. In the UK, there are more cases of basal cell carcinoma than all other types (skin and non-skin) of cancer put together. Malignant melanoma is less common with an incidence in a similar population of about 10–15 per 100 000.

12.3 Is skin cancer just a problem in old age?

No, but skin cancer is much commoner in the elderly. Skin cancer can occur in children and young adults and, when it does, it is always worth looking for a special reason. Reasons can include inherited conditions such as xeroderma pigmentosum (*see* Q 12.7) and Gorlin's syndrome (*see* Q 12.8), immunosuppression (e.g. in a transplant recipient) and with excessive ultraviolet (UV) exposure (e.g. in a sunbed addict).

12.4 Is skin cancer serious – do people die from it?

This question is best dealt with by limiting the answer to the three most commonly diagnosed skin cancers – basal cell carcinoma, squamous cell carcinoma and malignant melanoma. Although the other types of skin cancer contain some notoriously lethal tumours such as Merkel cell and sebaceous carcinomas, they are rare.

> Basal cell carcinoma is rarely fatal. It does not spread but erodes through underlying tissue so potentially fatal problems only occur if the tumour is neglected and penetrates the skull or a major blood vessel. Squamous cell carcinoma does kill people more commonly as around 1–2% of cases will metastasize. Malignant melanomas are more likely to be fatal, the prognosis being worse the thicker the tumour is at presentation. For patients with a melanoma less than 1 mm thick, the likelihood of death due to the disease is only about 10% but this rises to about 30% for a tumour with a thickness of 3 mm.

12.5 Is there a premalignant phase when cancer could be prevented?

Yes, for squamous cell carcinomas and some types of malignant melanoma. The former often begins as an actinic keratosis or Bowen's disease. These lesions have the potential to become malignant as they have within them cells with the same abnormalities that are seen in squamous cell carcinomas. The difference is that the abnormal cells are confined to the epidermis and the cancer proper only develops once the cells have penetrated into the dermis. This process may take years.

Hutchinson's freckle, also known as lentigo maligna (LM), is a premalignant condition from which malignant melanoma can arise. This is seen on the face or other exposed skin sites in the elderly as an irregular pigmented macule which may have been slowly enlarging for years. When it transforms, an invasive nodule is seen and the name changes to lentigo maligna melanoma (LMM).

12.6 Are some people more at risk of developing skin cancer?

> Yes. The risk factors for most skin cancers can be classified as innate (inborn) or acquired (due to environmental factors) (*Box 12.1*). There may be some useful clues from examination, suggesting an increased susceptibility – for example, many actinic keratoses, patches of Bowen's disease or multiple, unusual-looking (dysplastic or atypical) moles.

GENETIC DISORDERS

12.7 What is xeroderma pigmentosum?

This is a name given to a heterogeneous collection of autosomal recessive disorders which are rare – affecting perhaps 5 per million in European

---

BOX 12.1 Risk factors for skin cancer

Innate
- Inherited syndromes – Gorlin's, xeroderma pigmentosum
- Familial melanoma
- Other cancer-prone disorders
- Skin type – fair skin, freckles, blue eyes

Acquired
- Ultraviolet exposure
- Immunosuppression, e.g. transplant recipient
- Viruses – some human papilloma viruses (SCC), human herpes virus 8 (Kaposi's)
- Arsenic ingestion
- Ionising radiation
- Tar/pitch exposure
- Chronic ulcers and scars

---

populations. The genetic abnormality leads to problems with the repair of DNA after it has been damaged by UV radiation. Affected infants soon develop photosensitivity and signs of sun damage soon appear in the form of freckles and actinic keratoses. These are soon followed by all three of the main types of skin cancer. Strict sun avoidance is needed but the severest forms of the condition usually prove fatal in the second and third decades.

12.8 Is Gorlin's syndrome common?

No it is quite rare. It is also caused by a genetic abnormality – recently shown to be on chromosome 9q – inherited as an autosomal dominant trait with some variable penetrance. Another name for it gives more of a clue as to the problems caused – the naevoid basal cell carcinoma syndrome. Patients show other anomalies such as abnormalities of the skull, vertebrae and ribs, jaw cysts and palmoplantar pits. Having the syndrome gives a lifetime chance of developing a basal cell carcinoma of 50% and lesions are often multiple.

12.9 What is meant by 'familial melanoma'?

This term has recently been introduced to typify both families with atypical moles and a tendency to develop melanomas, and those without moles but melanomas occurring in several members of succesive generations.

Atypical moles are multiple, large, irregular and variably pigmented naevi. They are most noticeable on the trunk but may occur in unusual places such as the scalp and the soles. They can be over 1 cm in diameter and may number in the hundreds. They can affect only one family member but more commonly occur through several generations as an autosomal dominant trait. Not all families have the same risk of melanoma – some have had a 'melanoma' gene identified on chromosomes 1p36 and 9p13 and there may well be other genes to be identified.

Patients with atypical moles and a family history of melanoma should be considered to be in the 'familial melanoma' classification and should be regularly reviewed – every 6 months – in the hope of detecting melanoma at an early and less invasive stage.

ACTINIC KERATOSIS

12.10 How do you spot an actinic keratosis?

Actinic keratoses (sometimes referred to as solar keratoses) occur on the most sun-exposed sites – the face, scalp (if bald) and backs of the hands. There is usually a yellowish or brown area of keratinous material with an underlying red base but sometimes only the red base. Actinic keratoses are typically harder to the touch than seborrhoeic keratoses and, unlike squamous cell carcinomas, there is no induration at the base when it is felt between finger and thumb.

12.11 Can actinic keratoses be managed in primary care?

'Management' implies considering both the lesion and the patient. The diagnosis of an actinic keratosis should lead to a thorough examination of the skin to search for other lesions and skin cancer. This should be combined with education about the effects of UV exposure and advice about sun protection for the future.

Most actinic keratoses are actually benign and remain so – only about one in a thousand lesions per year evolve into squamous cell carcinomas. Treatment may, therefore, just be indicated because lesions are unsightly, bleed with slight trauma, itch or are uncomfortable. All will benefit from a good emollient regimen to minimize scaling and dryness, which may be enough for many patients if it makes the lesions less obvious and less itchy.

For single or few lesions, the options in primary care include liquid nitrogen cryotherapy and curettage. If there are large, ill-defined or numerous lesions, application of 5% fluorouracil cream (Efudix) or diclofenac gel (Solaraze) can be effective. The former is more irritant but can result in clearance more quickly than the latter. Topical imiquimod has also recently shown some promise.

If there is uncertainty about whether the lesion is an actinic keratosis or an early squamous cell carcinoma, excision has the advantage of generating a sample for histology. It could also be curative if cancer was found which is less likely to be the case if the lesion were simply curetted off.

BOWEN'S DISEASE

12.12 Is Bowen's disease similar to actinic keratosis?

Like actinic keratosis, Bowen's disease presents as a red lesion with some degree of overlying hyperkeratosis. An individual lesion is likely to grow much larger than an actinic keratosis and becomes large enough to be referred to as a plaque. There is also a difference in the degree of likelihood of progression to skin cancer: in Bowen's disease, the malignant-looking cells are distributed throughout the full thickness of the epidermis whereas, in actinic keratoses, they are only found in the lower part. Each lesion of Bowen's disease has a greater likelihood of evolving into squamous cell carcinoma, and is also referred to as an intraepidermal carcinoma.

12.13 How should Bowen's disease be managed?

Bowen's disease can be left alone and observed for likely evolution into squamous cell carcinoma but this should only be an option for the frail or very elderly unless chosen by a suitably well-informed patient. Several treatments lead to an acceptable level of cure. These include 5% fluorouracil cream, imiquimod cream, liquid nitrogen cryotherapy, curettage and electrodesiccation, photodynamic therapy and excision with appropriate repair. The choice will depend on size, site, availability of the treatment locally, and the ability of the patient to cope with the likely consequences.

12.14 What are the risks if Bowen's disease is left untreated?

Patches of Bowen's disease grow slowly and are usually asymptomatic. The larger they grow, the more morbidity there can be if treatment is eventually used. They often occur on areas with little laxity in the skin (e.g. the shin) and closure after excision can be difficult even with small lesions. A small percentage will evolve into squamous cell carcinomas (about 3% over 10 years) but there is a dearth of data to confirm this.

BASAL CELL CARCINOMA

12.15 Do basal cell carcinomas spread?

In the sense of distant spread, the simplest answer is no. Metastases from basal cell carcinomas (BCCs) have been reported in patients with advanced, neglected, destructive tumours around the mouth and nose who inhale fragments of BCC which then settle and grow in the lungs. There are some well-documented cases of true metastasis via the lymphatics but these are so rare that most dermatologists will never see a case. BCCs do spread locally and this can sometimes have devastating effects as when the skull or major blood vessels are invaded in badly neglected cases.

12.16 Should basal cell carcinomas be managed differently for different presentations?

Basal cell carcinomas can vary greatly in both pattern and speed of growth. The choice of treatment will depend on many factors including the type of BCC, the site and the general health and age of the patient. The common growth patterns are:

- exophytic – grows mainly outwards as a semi-translucent nodule
- endophytic – grows inwards; these ulcerate early and can become deeply invasive
- superficial – spread as a patch with a slightly raised border; seen most often on the trunk
- morpheic – an ill-defined indurated plaque.

Sites where BCCs can be harder to cure and are potentially more dangerous include on and beside the nose, around the eyes and the ears. For most invasive BCCs, the best option is excision with appropriate repair. Radiotherapy may be preferable for some inoperable cases. Selected superficial BCCs, and some small BCCs of other types at less important sites, can be treated effectively with curettage and electrodesiccation. This technique can also be used for other superficial BCCs but there are other options such as photodynamic therapy, liquid nitrogen cryotherapy or the topical creams 5% fluorouracil and imiquimod. Apart from curettage, where material is available for histological confirmation of the diagnosis, these methods destroy the lesion without the possibility of confirming the diagnosis so doctors treating patients must be certain of the diagnosis on clinical grounds. For some large superficial BCCs a small punch biopsy could be taken for histology prior to the destructive treatment.

For some large deep primary BCCs, and some recurrent cases at critical sites, a technique known as Mohs' surgery should be considered. This involves progressive removal of the tumour and histological assessment of the deep margins – usually from a frozen section – while the patient waits, until no further tumour is found.

12.17 How much follow-up is needed?

Follow-up is appropriate in three different circumstances:

- if it is uncertain that a BCC has been cured
- if it is likely that the patient will develop new skin cancer and that self-examination will not be a reliable enough way of detecting this

- to judge the cosmetic and/or functional consequences of treatment.

If a BCC has been excised, and the histologist confirms that this is complete, recurrence is highly unlikely. When other modalities of treatment are used it may not be possible for the histologist to report on totality of excision (curettage), or there may not be any sampled tissue (cryotherapy/creams), and it is therefore prudent to inspect the treated area for the possibility of recurrence.

BCC can grow very slowly and recurrence may not be evident for years so it is very helpful when the patients and their nearest-and-dearest can play an effective role in detecting possible recurrences. Some individuals develop new skin cancers during follow-up, justifying a planned visit to the doctor at intervals of, perhaps, a few months to not only inspect sites of previous treatment, but also to examine for any new cancer or pre-cancer.

SQUAMOUS CELL CARCINOMA

12.18 Are squamous cell carcinomas more dangerous than basal cell carcinomas?

Yes. Squamous cell carcinoma (SCC) can metastasize and, when this happens, death from the disease is quite likely. Although SCC arising after chronic UV exposure is unlikely to metastasize – perhaps only 3% risk – certain sites are more dangerous, notably the lower lip, the ear and non-sun-exposed sites such as the perineum. Aggressive behaviour is also associated with large and deeply invasive tumours, growth around nerves (perineural spread), poor histological differentiation, and aetiology other than from UV (chronic ulcer or sinus) and in the immunosuppressed.

12.19 Is it safe to do a biopsy?

Yes. Appropriate management requires a tissue diagnosis and with many tumours this will only come from the histologist. An incisional biopsy is appropriate for a tumour that cannot be easily excised, especially if the diagnosis is not apparent clinically. Even with melanoma, the prognosis is not adversely affected by an incisional biopsy.

12.20 Should squamous cell carcinomas be managed in centres of excellence only?

It is reasonable to treat some SCCs in primary care if there are the skills and facilities to do so. There should also be links with secondary care services so that guidelines about management and follow-up are standardized throughout a locality. In the UK, the National Institute for Clinical Excellence advises that anyone managing skin cancer should be part of a local multidisciplinary team or network. If a small, low-risk SCC can be excised with a 4 mm margin and sent for histology, current standards of surgical treatment will have been met but overall management also requires guidelines for diagnosis, time to treatment and follow-up.

For the higher risk SCC, it is likely that referral to secondary care would be best practice.

MALIGNANT MELANOMA

12.21 How can GPs minimize the risk of missing a malignant melanoma?

There is no substitute for experience and training but four rules can help minimize the risk of missing a melanoma or failing to refer to someone who might be better placed to make or exclude the diagnosis.

■ Always keep the possibility that a lesion could be a melanoma somewhere in your differential diagnosis.
■ Remember that melanomas are not always pigmented.
■ Encourage patients to come back if they are concerned about continuing growth in a lesion that worries them even if you are confident on current history and clinical examination that it is benign.
■ Take every opportunity to look at *all* the skin; some 'missed melanomas' are those the patient has not noticed.

12.22 Should all suspected melanomas be referred to a specialist?

Yes. The current UK guidelines on management of malignant melanoma (MM) specify that a patient with a suspected MM should be referred urgently to a dermatologist or plastic surgeon. 'Urgently' equates to no more than 2 weeks between the visits to the GP and to the specialist. The same should apply to any patient in whom a biopsy, whether incisional or excisional, of a harmless-looking lesion is reported by the histologist as MM.

12.23 Are acral melanomas more likely to spread?

Location of a melanoma on the extremities is a poor prognostic pointer. This may be because plantar and subungual melanomas have often attained a dangerous degree of thickness before they are diagnosed.

12.24 Is it OK to observe a lentigo maligna without treatment in a frail old person?

It depends on the circumstances! If the LM can be excised with a 0.5–1 cm margin and the defect repaired relatively easily, this is preferable. The likelihood of evolution to LMM is quite low, so for an 80-year-old it might only represent a lifetime risk of 5%. If the size of the lesion and/or the co-morbidities are such that surgery would be risky or leave the patient with a significant problem, then it is reasonable to observe and only intervene if there is clinical suspicion that a melanoma is developing. There may be the possibility in the future that a topical treatment could be used to avoid surgery in frail patients.

12.25 Do any of the common cancers present with a metastasis on the skin?

Metastases occurring in the skin are occasionally the first indication of an internal cancer, but they more commonly occur after the primary has been diagnosed. They most often involve a site somewhere near the primary tumour (e.g. in the umbilical region for a variety of intestinal cancers). For several cancers the scalp is a relatively common distant site – notably for renal, thyroid and breast tumours – and this can present as a patch of alopecia.

The most common primary internal cancers to metastasize to the rest of the skin in males are from the lung, large intestine and oral cavity. In females breast is much the commonest, followed by large intestine and ovary. It must not be forgotten that melanoma can metastasize to the skin and that the initial presentation may be a metastasis rather than the primary – sometimes after failure to send an apparently benign excised lesion for histological examination.

 PATIENT QUESTIONS

12.26 Will getting a tan protect me from skin cancer?

No. Although darker skin does offer some added sun protection this is only equivalent to about a sun protection factor of 2. This means that you will get just as much damage from the sun but it will take twice as much time. You will actually tend to spend longer in the sun as you will not get the same burning sensation or be likely to go as red. A tan can, therefore, give you a very false sense of security.

12.27 I have had a rodent ulcer removed – what are my chances of getting another one?

Rodent ulcers, called basal cell cancers by doctors, are the result of long-term, low level exposure to sunlight or other sources of UV radiation. They are, therefore, often a problem for people who have worked outdoors or have hobbies or sports that take place in the open air. Examples would be the building trade, gardening, golf and sailing. All of your skin that has been exposed will have an increased chance of developing another rodent ulcer but it is impossible to give you an absolute risk. You will need to be vigilant and look out for any new changes on your skin and to seek medical advice for anything you are suspicious of.

12.28 I try to avoid getting too much sun but do like my 2 week holiday on a foreign beach every year. Is this still risky?

Yes, it is. Long-term exposure is linked to basal and squamous cell cancers but the sort of exposure you describe is much more closely linked to malignant melanoma – the most dangerous type of cancer. Pale skin and a desire to get as much sun as possible in a short space of time is very risky as you will probably burn quite a bit in the first few days. You can still have your holiday and come home with your tan if you avoid the strongest sun, use sunscreen and a shade on the beach, wear a hat and clothing thick enough or coloured enough to block out the UV when you are out and about.

Drug reactions and rashes
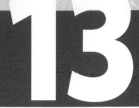

13

13.1 Almost every drug seems to have 'skin rashes' listed as a possible side effect in the data sheet. Is this a real problem?

Yes, both prescribed and self-medicated drugs are a major cause of skin disease, sometimes serious and occasionally life threatening (e.g. toxic epidermal necrolysis). Many skin diseases can be mimicked by a reaction to drugs – for example, eczema, lichen planus and rashes due to viral infection. Some naturally occurring skin diseases can be brought on or worsened by a drug (e.g. psoriasis exacerbated by lithium or chloroquine). If a person has developed contact allergy to a chemical and takes a drug which is chemically similar, a widespread eczema may occur.

13.2 Why do drugs give rise to skin rashes?

There are many different ways in which drug reactions are caused. Both the properties of the individual drugs and the susceptibility of patients are important. The mechanisms of reaction can be divided into two broad groups: non-allergic and allergic (*Box 13.1*).

13.3 Are non-allergic drug reactions common?

Yes, you only have to look at the lists of possible side effects in any drug formulary to see that many drugs seem capable of producing skin rashes even

---

BOX 13.1 Mechanisms of drug reaction

Non-allergic
- Pharmacological, e.g. striae and acne from corticosteroids, dry lips from isotretinoin, mouth ulcers from cytotoxics
- Toxic effects from higher than normal therapeutic levels due to overdosage or problems with excretion or metabolism, e.g. purpura from warfarin overdosage
- Cumulative effects, e.g. deposition of drug in the skin from gold- or silver-based products
- Effect on normal skin flora, e.g. candidiasis after antibiotics
- Worsening of existing condition, e.g. psoriasis with beta-blockers or lithium
- Idiosyncratic reactions peculiar to an individual

Allergic from any of the four types of immune hypersensitivity
- IgE mediated
- Immune complex reactions
- Cell mediated
- Humoral cytotoxic

if only at the higher doses used in initial testing. Some reactions are predictable, especially those listed in Box 13.1 as pharmacological, toxic, cumulative and worsening of an existing condition. Many skin reactions are, however, unpredictable and with no known mechanism so they are labelled as idiosyncratic – for want of a better word. These are also very common.

13.4 Can allergic reactions be predicted?

Not really. They affect only a small proportion of the patients taking a particular drug. The reaction can come on at low doses but after the usual latent period for the immune response to develop. Allergic reactions can present in many different ways but the common ones are urticaria and angioedema, vasculitis, erythema multiforme and morbilliform eruptions.

Rarer presentations include bullae, erythroderma, pruritus and toxic epidermal necrolysis.

13.5 What is the hypersensitivity syndrome reaction?

This is a term used to group together some of the more serious reactions involving a systemic response. There is usually a triad of fever, rash and internal involvement. The rash can vary from morbilliform to exfoliative dermatitis and the internal involvement can lead to haematological problems, nephritis, hepatitis and pneumonitis.

13.6 When should a drug reaction be suspected?

Any unusual rash should trigger suspicions, especially in older patients on multiple medications. Always remember to ask about over-the-counter preparations bought without a prescription. There are different points to consider once your suspicions have been raised.

- Has a straightforward skin disease or the skin signs of an underlying medical problem been excluded?
- Is the rash typical of a drug reaction?
- Has the patient had a previous drug reaction and are any related (or the same!) drugs being prescribed?
- Does the current prescription include drugs that commonly cause reactions?

13.7 What are the common types of reaction and the drugs most likely to be involved?

This is set out in *Table 13.1* which is by no means complete! More details of the different types of reaction are given in other chapters.

TABLE 13.1 Drug reactions

Reaction	Appearances	Drug example
Exanthem	Resembles viral infection, e.g. measles	Amoxicillin, carbamazepine
Urticaria and anaphylaxis	Weals, i.e. like nettle rash	Penicillin, vaccines
Exfoliative dermatitis	Generalized redness and scaling	Gold
Purpura	Flat, non-blanching purple patches	Cytotoxic drugs, thiazides
Erythema multiforme	Target lesions on extremities	Antibiotics, anticonvulsants
Stevens–Johnson syndrome (SJS)	Ulcers on the mucosa of the mouth, genital area and eyes	
Toxic epidermal necrolysis	Widespread tender rash which blisters, mucosal changes like SJS	
Lichenoid eruption	Purplish-red flat-topped shiny lesions	Diuretics, antimalarials, NSAIDs
Bullous	Blisters, e.g. resembling porphyria	NSAIDs
Acne-like	Spots resembling acne	Corticosteroids, lithium, oral contraceptives
Vasculitis	Non-blanching purple spots; some may form ulcers	Antibiotics, phenytoin, indometacin, oral contraceptives
Fixed eruption	Episodes of inflammation, sometimes with a blister, at the same site each time, followed by increased pigmentation	Paracetamol, NSAIDs, tetracycline, psychotropic drugs
Pigmentation	Brown, grey or bluish patches	Minocycline, antimalarials
Hair loss	Diffuse over the scalp	Acitretin, cytotoxics, anticoagulants, oral contraceptives
Excess hair growth	Affects vellus hair	Minoxidil, phenytoin, corticosteroids, ciclosporin
Phototoxic	Usually resembles sunburn	Thiazides, amiodarone, NSAIDs, phenothiazines

NSAIDs, non-steroidal anti-inflammatory drugs.

13.8 What is a fixed drug eruption?

As noted in *Table 13.1*, this is a reaction that occurs each time the offending drug is taken and presents at the site of the previous reaction. It usually presents as a round, red or purple thin plaque which can blister. As it resolves, post-inflammatory hyperpigmentation is left which persists until the next episode. The reaction can occur on any part of the skin including the glans penis which may, in fact, be one of the commoner sites. Paracetamol is the commonest culprit in the UK – underlining the need for a careful history of over-the-counter medications.

13.9 How should drug reactions be managed?

The symptomatic treatment will vary according to the type of reaction seen, but the obvious approach is to identify and withdraw the drug that is causing it. Assessment of the whole patient, and including the patient in the decision-making process, is needed to weigh up the balance between the problem caused by the reaction, the need for the drug and the availability of any alternatives. There are no reliable tests to identify the particular drug so careful attention must be given to the history of the reaction and any link to the introduction of new medications.

13.10 Can patients be desensitized?

This is sometimes possible and necessary under specialist supervision. It applies only when essential drugs are involved with no alternatives available. These rare indications include anticonvulsants and antituberculous therapy.

13.11 What is the treatment of anaphylaxis?

This is a medical emergency so basic principles of life support apply, including maintenance of an airway. This may need a tracheostomy in the case of gross pharyngeal oedema.

Adrenaline (1:1000) should be given either subcutaneously or intramuscularly – 0.3–0.5 ml in adults – and repeated if necessary. Chlorpheniramine is the most common antihistamine recommended and needs to be given as a slow intravenous injection of 10–20 mg over 1 minute; 10 ml of blood can be drawn back into the syringe at the start to facilitate this slow injection.

A corticosteroid in the form of 100 mg hydrocortisone should also be given intravenously after the other drugs. It will have no immediate effect as its onset of action is not for several hours – it is given to prevent further deterioration in severe cases.

Patients should be kept under observation for about 6 hours after they have been stabilized. Those at risk of further attacks should be provided with adrenaline for self-administration and, perhaps, a salbutamol inhaler.

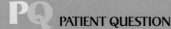 **PATIENT QUESTION**

13.12 If I react badly to one drug, am I more likely to react to another one?

It is a bit tricky to generalize. Some drugs are linked together by having a common origin or similar chemical structures and reacting to one of these should mean avoidance of some others. The best example of this is penicillin where one reaction means that you should avoid all penicillins (e.g. amoxicillin and flucloxacillin). The penicillins are also linked to another group of antibiotics called cephalosporins so these should be avoided as well. Most GPs will have your reaction noted and the modern computer systems used will 'flag up' the reaction when the doctor looks at your notes.

Other than this situation, one reaction does not mean you will be any more likely to have another reaction to a different drug.

Foreign travel

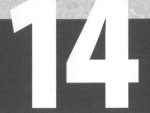

14

14.1 Why does foreign travel merit a mention in this book?

Knowing that a patient has ventured abroad can offer important new areas of possible diagnoses for a presenting clinical problem, or help explain an ongoing one. The foreign travel may have led to extremes of climate, noxious animal or plant life, infectious agents not found in the homeland or risky, disinhibited behaviour.

14.2 What can happen to existing skin problems in different climates?

- Acne may temporarily improve with ultraviolet (UV) exposure but usually worsens if conditions are hot and humid. Patients on tetracyclines will be at risk of problems from phototoxicity.
- Atopic eczema also sometimes improves with UV but secondary infection can be a problem in hot, humid conditions.
- Although psoriasis generally improves with UV exposure, it can worsen and patients should avoid chloroquine-based antimalarials which can trigger a flare.
- UV exposure may also worsen diseases like lupus erythematosus, porphyrias and photodermatoses and can trigger herpes simplex.
- Cold conditions rarely cause problems for existing skin conditions but can cause problems for patients with cryoglobulinaemia who would be at risk of purpura, urticaria and livedo reticularis.

14.3 Is it just the different conditions abroad that cause problems or is it also different behaviour?

It depends on the circumstances. For example, it may be that the strength of the UV is no greater but the person on holiday will spend more time exposed to it. Behavioural changes are also important in contracting diseases that might not be a problem at home. Syphilis is one example where behaviour on holiday could be much less inhibited than it would be at home. Human immunodeficiency virus (HIV) infection is also a risk but much less likely to give rise to skin problems in the short term.

14.4 Are there any clues from history or examination that might prompt a question about foreign travel?

As already noted, worsening of a pre-existing dermatosis could be due to climatic change. Any unexplained and unusual skin disease might just be a consequence of an exposure or event while the patient was abroad which is why foreign travel is an important part of routine history taking for skin disease. The patient may not have made the connection in conditions where there is a latent period so might not volunteer the information. Examples here would be cutaneous leishmaniasis and larva migrans.

14.5 Are foreign fungal infections more difficult to manage?

Fungal infections presenting in the skin can be broadly classified as superficial, subcutaneous and systemic. Infections contracted abroad may well be from the same species that will be encountered in the UK (e.g. *Trichophyton rubrum* and *Candida albicans*) but there are some species that are only found overseas. Although these will rarely cause serious problems, the treatment can depend on exactly what fungus is causing the problem so specialist mycology laboratories must be used as they will have the expertise to isolate and identify exotic species. *Table 14.1* summarizes the more common problems.

14.6 Do insect-borne diseases present with skin problems?

Insects and arthropods (ticks, mites and spiders) are responsible for transmitting a wide variety of diseases that manifest in the skin – and many that do not such as malaria. Insects can also cause troublesome lesions directly (e.g. bites from bed bugs) and when the larval form parasitizes skin (e.g. myiasis and tungiasis).

The incubation period may be just a few days as in dengue (fever, widespread haemorrhagic rash and bone pain), weeks to months as in leishmaniasis (non-healing sores), or even longer as with some of the itchy eruptions due to parasitic worms, onchocerciasis and loiasis.

14.7 What is myiasis?

Cutaneous myiasis occurs when the larvae of dipteran flies develop in the skin. Some species of fly require larval development in living skin and it is an encounter with one of these that may produce the distinctive lesions. Myiasis may also occur when eggs are laid in an existing wound and a wider variety of fly larvae can thrive in such circumstances. The flies whose larvae are able to penetrate intact skin generally utilize a mammal other than man as their preferred primary host. In Africa, the commonest is the tumbu fly (*Cordylobia anthropophaga*) and in the New World the likely culprits are the human botfly (*Dermatobium hominis*) and the screw worm (*Cochliomya hominivorax*).

How the larvae get into human skin varies with the species. *D. hominis* is unique in having the ability of hitching a ride with a mosquito, myiasis

TABLE 14.1 Examples of exotic fungal infections

Classification	Disease	Description	Treatment
Superficial	Tinea nigra	Brown patch, usually on palm	Topical azole
	Piedra	Coloured nodules on hair shafts	Shave off affected hair
	Scytalidium infection	Resembles tinea of hands, feet and nails but fungus will not grow on standard media – thus often reported as 'fungus seen but not grown'	Sometimes responds to tioconazole
	Favus	Usually distinctive type of tinea capitis with cup-shaped, yellowish crusts	Longer course of oral antifungal
Subcutaneous	Sporotrichosis	Nodules and ulcers along route of lymphatic drainage	Oral potassium iodide, itraconazole or IV amphotericin B
	Mycetoma	Destructive soft tissue infection with abscesses and discharge of 'grains'	Depends on species
	Chromoblastomycosis	Warty plaques and nodules, subcutaneous swellings ± lymphoedema, depending on disease and causative fungus	Depends on species
	Phaeohyphomycosis		
	Lobomycosis		
	Zygomycosis		
Systemic	Histoplasmosis	Papules, nodules and ulcers in the setting of a generalized illness	Depends on species
	Blastomycosis		
	Coccidioidomycosis	Respiratory illness; erythema nodosum common	Itraconazole, amphotericin B
	Paracoccidioidomycosis	Mucocutaneous granulomatous nodules	
	Cryptococcosis	Papules, nodules and pustules	IV amphotericin B

being added to the list of miseries inflicted on humans by this insect. The lesions are on exposed parts and resemble boils. There is a central punctum, through which the posterior breathing end of the maggot protrudes and can sometimes be seen to move.

14.8 How is myiasis treated?

Most of the maggot is below the surface and its body has backward pointing spikes that make it very difficult to pull the creature out intact. The trick is to cut off the air supply which can be done by smothering the lesion in petroleum jelly. More of the body will then emerge, making complete extraction easier. Sometimes a cruciate incision to enlarge the punctum will still be necessary.

14.9 Can cutaneous larva migrans be treated in the same way?

Cutaneous larva migrans is most commonly caused by the larval form of a dog hookworm. Rare causes include the larvae of certain flies (Gasterophilus and Hypoderma) but this answer applies only to the hookworm variety. The typical location for acquiring dog hookworm is from a sandy shore where dogs defaecate. The feet, buttocks and hands are, therefore, the commonest sites for lesions. There may be an interval of as long as several months before the characteristic itchy, wandering track-like lesion(s) are first seen. Although it tends to be self-limiting, it can last several months and a number of treatments are effective. Probably the best are a single dose of ivermectin (200 mcg/kg) or albendazole (400 mg/day for 3 days).

14.10 Can fleas cause problems?

Worldwide, fleas are a common source of itchy bite reactions, the most common being cat or dog fleas, and, in communities where there is poor hygiene, human fleas. The lesions vary and can include papules, nodules and bullae, grouped together or in a linear distribution. A particular problem for the foreign traveller is the sand flea, *Tunga penetrans*. This tiny flea can penetrate the skin, usually between the toes, and cause a growing itching nodule. The condition is sometimes known as jiggers and may need to be debrided or excised.

14.11 What is the result of stepping on a sea urchin?

Sea urchins can produce deep penetrating wounds because of their very sharp calcified spines, which can break off and remain embedded, and their pedicellaria (jaw-like structures) in amongst the spines. In some species they can transmit venom which causes extreme pain and sometimes paraesthesia and even paralysis. They can also introduce infection, with tetanus being a significant hazard because of the depth of the wound.

Penetration of the calcified spines can damage joints and neurovascular bundles and, if this is likely, appropriate surgical care is needed although many cases of minor injury settle spontaneously. Sometimes granulomatous nodules can persist in the long term and may need to be x-rayed to identify the calcific material as the cause. Intralesional steroid injections may help some lesions.

14.12 Is there a difference between 'seabather's eruption' and 'swimmer's itch'?

These are both itchy papular conditions, but the distribution and causes differ. Both can last 1–2 weeks.

- Seabather's eruption is a hypersensitivity reaction to thimble jellyfish larvae and occurs beneath bathing costumes. It is common off the Florida coast. Fever, malaise, abdominal pain and other systemic symptoms accompany the intense itching.
- Swimmer's itch – also known as schistosome cercarial dermatitis – is due to a hypersensitivity reaction to non-human (often bird) schistosome larvae. It has a worldwide distribution and occurs mainly after bathing in fresh water but has been reported from some saltwater lagoons. The skin under bathing costumes is protected and the itching comes on rapidly. Systemic symptoms are uncommon.

Treatment for both conditions is symptomatic with antihistamines, soothing creams and occasionally topical steroids. Prevention for seabather's eruption can be helped by removing costumes and showering immediately and for swimmer's itch by towelling dry immediately after leaving the water as the larvae seem to penetrate the skin as the water is evaporating from the skin.

14.13 Why are some jellyfish stings so serious?

Jellyfish tentacles have specialized cells called nematocysts which can deliver venom via a coiled, sharpened hollow tube. The venom can cause both toxic and allergic reactions. Although most instances of contact with jellyfish produce no more than mildly unpleasant reactions, some species are associated with severe pain. The best known of these is the Portuguese Man-of-War but despite the serious sounding name it is not the worst species to encounter. Some stings have an appreciable mortality such as the Pacific box jellyfish found off the coast of Australia. A lethal dose of its toxin is only 40 mcg/kg. As well as death, serious sequelae include major vessel thrombosis, extensive skin necrosis and serious eye injury.

14.14 What is the best treatment for a jellyfish sting?

It is very important to have a reasonable idea of what type of jellyfish has produced the injury. Local knowledge of the varieties found, a description of the jellyfish (if possible) and the pattern of sting reactions can all help. Treatment can include all or some of the following:

- Deactivation of nematocysts – rinsing with sterile saline; soaking with vinegar, for the Pacific box jellyfish; careful removal of tentacles
- Pain control with ice packs and analgesics
- Local wound care as appropriate
- Symptomatic treatment, e.g. antihistamine, corticosteroid
- Vital organ support
- Antivenom – for some box jellyfish stings
- Prevention of further problems – tetanus booster and treatment of secondary infection.

 PATIENT QUESTIONS

14.15 Why do some people seem to suffer much more from insect bites than others?

There are probably several factors that lead to this. An insect bite produces an initial stab sensation and then a delayed reaction to the tiny amounts of saliva left behind in the skin. Some people are much more sensitive to the saliva and react much more strongly with red lumps and sometimes blisters. The more bites suffered, the more likely that a strong reaction will develop. Hypersensitivity can lead to a widespread bumpy eruption referred to as 'papular urticaria'.

The immune system can become primed to react to bites so in some cases – mainly with mosquito bites – one new bite will lead to a flare-up at the sites of old bites.

It also seems that some people are unlucky enough to be more attractive to insects than others. This is probably due to differences in body odour that are not apparent to humans.

14.16 What is the best way to treat mosquito bites?

This depends on the severity of the reaction. A cream containing crotamiton at a strength of 10% in an emollient base (Eurax) can help, as can calamine lotion. An antihistamine tablet can be useful for bad reactions – either a non-sedative one during the day or a sedative one to reduce itching at night (or both). If the bites are badly scratched and become infected, medical advice should be sought in case antibiotics are needed. Frequent travellers often have their own favourite remedies and local knowledge may suggest a different approach.

14.17 Are there any vaccinations I should have to avoid skin problems abroad?

None of the common reactions discussed above can be avoided by vaccination – try to avoid the causes! There are often some vaccinations you should have for other diseases, including yellow fever which is spread by mosquitoes in some parts of Africa and South America.

Miscellaneous skin disorders

15

15.1 Can the skin give clues about systemic disease?

We learn as much about systemic disease from the skin as from any other organ system. Obvious examples include anaemia, heart failure, jaundice, uraemia, thyroid disease and AIDS. Many of the conditions discussed in this book are a prompt to look for a systemic disease – for example, erythema nodosum, vasculitis and pyoderma gangrenosum. The skin is so often the mirror in which we see hallmarks of a serious infection, such as the distinctive lesions of meningococcal septicaemia. Structural alterations of the skin as seen in diseases such as Ehlers–Danlos syndrome and pseudoxanthoma elasticum can be far more important internally as in the potentially fatal cardiovascular manifestations of these diseases. Pigmentary change may be an important clue to many systemic diseases – for example, the addisonian pattern of hyperpigmentation in palmar creases, oral mucosa and scars which occurs in both Addison's and Cushing's diseases.

Diffuse hyperpigmentation can be found in a diverse array of diseases including malabsorption and any wasting process. Internal malignancies occasionally present with a skin manifestation from direct involvement or a paraneoplastic phenomenon (*Box 15.1*).

Some distinctive lesions have a fairly high chance of being associated with particular systemic diseases such as necrobiosis lipoidica with diabetes mellitus and xanthomas with hyperlipidaemia. The autoimmune diseases systemic lupus erythematosus, dermatomyositis and scleroderma are usually recognized clinically by their distinctive cutaneous lesions.

BOX 15.1 Skin manifestations in systemic disease

- Acanthosis nigricans also with insulin resistance and occasionally as a drug eruption
- Dermatomyositis – consider malignancy in all but childhood cases
- Necrolytic migratory erythema – associated with glucagon-secreting tumour of the pancreas
- Paraneoplastic pemphigus
- Erythema gyratum repens
- Migratory superficial thrombophlebitis
- Acquired ichthyosis
- Acquired hypertrichosis lanuginosa
- Generalized pruritus

15.2 How common are skin changes in diabetes?

Many skin disorders can occur in diabetics but most are asymptomatic and probably not noticed unless looked for (*Box 15.2*). Diabetic dermopathy is said to occur in 50% of Type 1 diabetics but is rarely diagnosed. Some of the skin changes (e.g. necrobiosis lipoidica) raise a strong suspicion for diabetes mellitus either currently or in the future; most are much less specific (e.g. candidal infection).

Necrobiosis lipoidica (NL) occurs in less than 1% of diabetics but about 50% of those with NL have, or will develop, diabetes. The lesions are most common on the shins but can occur at many other sites. They are indurated, often purplish-brown in colour with depressed, shiny, yellowish centres over which there are usually telangiectatic blood vessels. Ulceration is a common complication.

Diabetic dermopathy mainly occurs over the shins, forearms, thighs and bony prominences. Initial lesions are dull red papules which gradually flatten, form a scale and settle, leaving a slightly atrophic brown mark.

Also rarely complained of is the cheiroarthropathy of Type 1 diabetes where there is a diffuse thickening of the skin and joints of the hands. This leads to the 'positive prayer sign', an inability to flatten out the fingers of one hand against the other. Scleroderma is one of several other diseases that can lead to the same changes.

Diabetic bullae are uncommon, arising from normal looking skin over the feet or lower legs.

BOX 15.2 Diabetes mellitus and skin changes

Skin changes	Strength of association with diabetes mellitus
Insulin-related reactions	++++
Diabetic dermopathy	++++
Necrobiosis lipoidica	+++
Diabetic bullae	+++
Granuloma annulare (generalized)	+
Neuropathic ulceration	+
Some infections, e.g. boils, Candida	+
Peripheral vascular disease and gangrene	+
Eruptive xanthomas	+
Scleredema	+

+ (weak) to ++++ (very strong).

15.3 Apart from good blood glucose control, are there any specific treatments for necrobiosis lipoidica?

Many treatments have been tried for necrobiosis lipoidica without much success. A potent topical steroid may have a useful effect on the advancing edge and, if not, it is worth trying an intralesional steroid injection.

15.4 Is granuloma annulare associated with diabetes?

In some circumstances! There has long been a reported association between generalized granuloma annulare (GA) and diabetes mellitus but some studies fail to confirm this. The localized form of GA with roughly annular groups of dermal nodules over the knuckles, elbows or dorsal foot is not associated.

15.5 Are there skin changes with thyroid disease?

The warm moist skin with palmar erythema of hyperthyroidism, and the pale, dry, yellowish skin of hypothyroidism are important but rather non-specific features that, in the context of other signs, are none the less useful clues. In both states there can be diffuse hair loss or generalized pruritus. It is worth noting that loss of the outer third of the eyebrow hair and asteatotic eczema, which have long been associated with hypothyroidism, are common in other circumstances.

More specific features are sometimes seen. Pretibial myxoedema – nodular plaques with a peau d'orange appearance – is seen in Graves' disease and occasionally in Hashimoto's thyroiditis. Thyroid acropachy – the combination of clubbing with soft tissue swelling and new bone formation affecting the ends of the digits – is seen in about 1% of patients with Graves' disease.

15.6 Why do patients with renal disease itch?

Pruritus, both localized and generalized, is common in patients with end stage renal disease but does not occur during acute renal failure and rarely improves with dialysis. The cause remains obscure because, although there may be a relationship with calcium, phosphate and parathormone levels, correction of these metabolic parameters rarely helps. These patients sometimes have dry skin and emollients are then of some value. Even though its mechanism is not understood, ultraviolet B (UVB) phototherapy is probably the most effective treatment modality.

15.7 Is pruritus the only skin problem in renal disease?

Many other skin problems can occur in patients with chronic renal disease. These include:

- dry skin
- pigmentary change – a general yellowish discoloration sometimes with hyperpigmentation on sun-exposed sites
- bullous disease – especially porphyria cutanea tarda
- calciphylaxis – a syndrome of vascular calcification and skin necrosis
- arterial steal syndrome – ischaemia in the hand distal to an arteriovenous fistula.

In patients who receive a transplanted kidney and are on immunosuppression there is an increased risk of skin malignancies, including Kaposi's sarcoma, opportunistic infections and treatment-related problems such as steroid acne.

15.8 What is pyoderma gangrenosum and what is it associated with?

Pyoderma gangrenosum (PG) is a primary ulcerative condition mediated by activated neutrophils. Typically, the initial presentation is an inflammatory nodule or deep pustule which breaks down to form an ulcer with a bluish edge. It is usually painful and can progressively enlarge both in area and depth. It is always important to exclude infection, vasculitis and sometimes other diseases that can resemble PG. Fifty per cent of cases are linked with a systemic disease such as ulcerative colitis, Crohn's disease, rheumatoid arthrtis, blood dyscrasias, monoclonal gammopathy and chronic liver disease. Patients should be referred to a specialist as large doses of corticosteroids are needed to treat it.

15.9 What are the most likely causes of pruritus without obvious skin disease?

Skin diseases that may have minimal or very subtle signs should be considered first. These include scabies and bullous pemphigoid where itching can precede the rash. In dermatitis herpetiformis the lesions may become so excoriated that the dominant physical sign is just scratch marks. Dry skin can also be the source of generalized pruritus in the elderly and some atopics itch with little or no visible eczema. Urticaria may be short lived, and so missed at examination.

Itching with no primary dermatological cause may be due to chronic renal failure, cholestatic liver disease, hyper- and hypothyroidism, occult malignancy (rare), possible iron deficiency and, usually by exclusion of other causes, psychological factors. A special, but distinctive, condition is aquagenic pruritus – itching on contact with water – which can be an important pointer to polycythaemia vera.

15.10 Which routine investigations are useful in a case of pruritus?

Do not simply do tests. A careful history and examination may well contribute more to the diagnosis. It is worth doing a full blood count, differential white cell count, ESR or plasma viscosity, ferritin, thyroid, liver and renal tests. A chest radiograph is probably the only imaging that should be done unless there are localizing abdominal or pelvic signs on examination. Occult blood tests and a midstream urine specimen complete the routine work-up. If no explanation is found and the pruritus persists, the process of full history, examination and screening should be repeated.

15.11 Apart from finding and treating a cause, what treatments are available for the relief of pruritus?

If there is dry skin, emollients are well worth trying. Menthol (0.5–1%) and crotamiton are often useful, if only for limited periods. A sedative antihistamine at night or low dose tricyclic antidepressant can sometimes help. If a systemic cause such as renal disease or polycythaemia is found, the pruritus can be alleviated by UVB phototherapy. The itch associated with cholestatic liver disease can be helped by the opioid antagonist naltrexone.

15.12 What is the best way to approach a complaint of hair loss?

Hair loss (alopecia) can be subdivided into diffuse and localized with a further distinction between scarring and non-scarring causes.

Diffuse hair loss is often unexplained but can occur as a result of chronic systemic illness, especially thyroid disorders, drug side effects (including oral contraceptives), iron deficiency and androgenetic balding. With localized loss, the differentiation between scarring and non-scarring causes becomes important as the patient will want to know the chances of regrowth (*Box 15.3*).

15.13 How should alopecia areata be managed?

Although there are a few cases where regrowth does not occur and some cases which keep relapsing, patients can be reassured that regrowth is the norm. The hair can look white or blond as it starts to regrow but goes back to its normal colour. The best 'treatment' may be to wear a wig but not many patients will want to do this.

> **BOX 15.3 Scarring and non-scarring causes of alopecia**
>
> **Scarring causes** (where there is permanent damage to hair follicles)
> - Kerion
> - Lichen planus
> - Lupus erythematosus
> - Sarcoidosis
> - Basal cell carcinoma
> - Burns and other trauma
>
> **Non-scarring causes**
> - Alopecia areata
> - Hair pulling or traction
> - Tinea capitis

Actual treatment is not guaranteed to work but patients may want to try it, depending on the extent of the hair loss. An intralesional steroid such as intradermal triamcinolone can lead to temporary regrowth but great care must be taken to avoid atrophy. Some dermatologists use a potent skin sensitizer – diphencyprone – to trigger an eczema and then use the lowest concentration to produce a mild erythema which does lead to regrowth. This may also be a temporary solution until natural regrowth takes over.

15.14 What are the common causes of erythroderma?

Erythroderma (exfoliative dermatitis) means that 90% or more of the skin is red with variable scaling. Common causes are eczema (all types), psoriasis, drug reaction, and leukaemia and lymphoma; rarer causes are pemphigus foliaceous and pityriasis rubra pilaris.

15.15 Are there ever any emergencies in dermatology?

Some infections which present with cutaneous signs are potentially fatal in less than 24 hours. These include meningococcal septicaemia, ecthyma gangrenosum (due to Pseudomonas septicaemia) and necrotizing fasciitis (*see* Q 6.10). Urticaria may presage anaphylaxis which is clearly an emergency. Angioedema, which may suggest C1 esterase inhibitor deficiency, can lead to life-threatening airway obstruction.

Some conditions presenting with purpura are also life threatening as in thrombocytopaenic purpura, disseminated intravascular coagulation and systemic vasculitis (*see* Q 8.12).

Under several different circumstances, the skin as an organ can fail leading to loss of heat, fluid, protein and electrolytes. The barrier function is also lost and this is accompanied by a massive outpouring of proinflammatory cytokines. Untreated, there is often progressive multiorgan failure. Because of the speed with which they occur, the most serious causes of skin failure are extensive thermal burns and toxic epidermal necrolysis. Less immediate but still serious are staphylococcal scalded skin syndrome (*see Q 6.11*), widespread autoimmune bullous disease and generalized pustular psoriasis (*see Q 4.7*). Although usually less dramatic, erythroderma can become an emergency, especially if there is cardiovascular compromise, hypothermia or sepsis.

 PATIENT QUESTION

15.16 I suffer badly from itching down below – on my vulva – and no cause has been found. Is there anything I can do to help?

Itching over the vulva (pruritus vulvae) and around the anus (pruritus ani) can be very distressing indeed. It often seems to lack an obvious cause and doctors often offer 'symptomatic' treatment with various creams or antihistamines. You can follow some simple rules to help minimize the problem.

- Try to avoid tight clothing made of materials that could irritate or cause sweating.
- Do not give in to the urge to scratch or rub, especially after going to the toilet
- Avoid soap, directly or indirectly, e.g. using bubble bath or lying in a bath after having washed your hair
- Use an emollient soap-free cleanser, e.g. aqueous cream, or just plain water
- If you don't have access to a bidet, consider buying a portable plastic one from a camping or caravanning shop. Gentle washing with warm water and the emollient is useful after using the toilet and if you have become very sweaty after exercise.

APPENDIX
Useful organizations and websites

GP and nurse information

All Party Parliamentary Group on Skin (APPGS)
3/19 Holmbush Road
London SW15 3LE
Tel: 0208 246 6428
Fax: 0208 789 0795

British Association of Dermatologists (BAD)
4 Fitzroy Square
London W1T 5HQ
Tel: 0207 383 0266
Fax: 0207 388 5263
Email: admin@bad.org.uk
www.bad.org.uk
BAD guidelines: www.bad.org.uk/doctors/guidelines
   Association of practising UK dermatologists who aim to continually improve the treatment and understanding of skin disease.

British Dermatological Nursing Group (BDNG)
4 Fitzroy Square
London W1T 5HQ
Tel: 0207 383 0266
Fax: 0207 388 5263
www.bdng.org.uk
   An independent speciality group for nurses and healthcare professionals with an interest in dermatology.

British Red Cross
UK Office
44 Moorfields
London EC2Y 9AL
Tel: 0870 170 7000
Fax: 020 7562 2000
www.redcross.org.uk
   For free advice and information on cosmetic camouflage to cover any skin condition, including acne scarring. Refers you to local branches.

Disfigurement Guidance Centre
PO Box 7
Cupar
Fife KY15 4PF
Fax: 01337 870310
www.skinlaserdirectory.org.uk
Produces annual directory listing private and NHS skin laser clinics; contains articles on latest research. Is freely available to health professionals or can be purchased for £5.00. No phone enquiries so please send SAE.

Primary Care Dermatology Society
Gable House
40 High Street
Rickmansworth WD3 1ER
Tel: 01923 711678
Fax: 01923 778131
Email: pcds@pcds.org.uk
www.pcds.org.uk
A forum where GPs can exchange views on primary care dermatology, develop skills and progress clinical research.

Research Council for Complementary Medicine
c/o 1 Harley Street
London W1G 9QD
Email: info@rccm.org.uk
www.rccm.org.uk
The aim of the RCCM is to develop and extend the evidence base for complementary medicine in order to provide practitioners and their patients with information about the effectiveness of individual therapies and the treatment of specific conditions.

Patient information
Acne Support Group
PO Box 9
Newquay TR9 6WG
Tel: 0870 870 2263
Email: alison@the-asg.demon.co.uk
www.stopspots.org; www.m2w3.com/acne
A registered charity that provides independent advice and support to anyone affected by acne or rosacea. Membership gives access to a range of information covering all aspects of acne.

Changing Faces
The Squire Centre
33–37 University Street
London WC1E 6JN
Tel: 0845 4500 275
Fax: 0845 4500 276
Email: info@changingfaces.org.uk
www.changingfaces.org.uk
A charity that helps people facially disfigured in any way to express themselves with more confidence, and combats many of their anxieties and negative feelings.

National Eczema Society
Hill House
Highgate Hill
London N19 5NA
Tel: 0207 281 3553
Fax: 0207 281 6395
Eczema Information Line: 0870 241 3604
Email: helpline@eczema.org
www.eczema.org
An organization dedicated to meeting the needs of people with eczema and their families.

Psoriasis Association
Milton House
7 Milton Street
Northampton NN2 7JG
Tel: 0845 676 0076 (calls charged at local rate)
Fax: 01604 792894
Email: mail@psoriasis.demon.co.uk
www.psoriasis-association.org.uk

Psoriatic Arthropathy Alliance
PO Box 111
St Albans AL2 3JQ
Tel: 0870 7703212
Fax: 0870 7703213
Email: info@paalliance.org
www.paalliance.org

Skin Care Campaign
Hill House
Highgate Hill
London N19 5NA
www.skincarecampaign.org
   An alliance of patient groups, health professionals and other organizations concerned with skincare. It campaigns for a better deal for people with a wide variety of skin problems. No enquiries from general public but a good website. Has links to other patient groups such as Acne Support Group, National Eczema Society, Psoriasis Association and Psoriatic Arthropathy Alliance (see above).

Skinship
Plascow Cottage
Kirkgunzeon
Dumfries DG2 8JT
Helpline: 01387 760567
www.ukselfhelp.info/skinship
   Provides information for people with any skin disorder.

Government sites and guidelines
- **Action on Dermatology** www.modern.nhs.uk/action-on
- **Department of Health** www.dh.gov.uk
- **Health & Safety Executive** www.hse.gov.uk
- **National Electronic Library for Health (NeLH)** (this is an excellent source, providing healthcare professionals and the public – through NHS Direct Online and the New Library Network – with knowledge and know-how to support healthcare-related decisions) www.library.nhs.uk/skin/
- **National Institute for Clinical Excellence (NICE)** (gives guidance on the use of treatments and disease management strategies; can also be accessed through NeLH) www.nice.org.uk
- **National Research Register (NRR)** (a database of ongoing and recently completed research projects funded by, or of interest to, the United Kingdom's National Health Service) www.nrr.nhs.uk

Informative websites
- www.bnf.org/bnf – Gives sound, up-to-date information on the use of medicines
- www.bsid.org.uk – Promotes research in dermatology
- www.bupa.co.uk/health_information – Fact sheets that can be downloaded
- www.dermatlas.org – A site with many different images of skin disease

- www.dermatology.co.uk – Dermatology.co.uk is an independent website providing an educational resource for skin conditions and their treatment to patients, the public and health professionals
- www.dermnetnz.org – Award-winning website of the New Zealand Dermatological Society; aims to provide authoritative information about the skin for health professionals and patients with skin diseases
- www.DermQuest.com – Another site with many images of skin disease
- www.google.com – then enter 'disease + emedicine' for the search
- www.gpnotebook.co.uk – Oxbridge Solutions is an encyclopaedia of medical information for GPs
- www.ifd.org – The International Foundation for Dermatology
- www.patient.co.uk – Patient UK medical search engine
- www.sign.ac.uk – The Scottish Intercollegiate Guidelines Network gives unbiased guidance on best medical practice through systematic evaluation of clinical evidence
- www.which.net/health/dtb – Website for the Drug and Therapeutics Bulletin which provides advice on treatments and patient notes

Journals

- http://bjd.manuscriptcentral.com – British Journal of Dermatology; need login and password to access site
- www.bmj.com – Online access to the BMJ
- www.thelancet.com – Worldwide electronic access to the journal content
- www.eblue.org – Journal of the American Academy of Dermatology; can also be accessed through the American Academy of Dermatology (AAD) website www.aad.org
- www.ebandolier.com – Guides evidence-based medicine through literature searches and summaries of meta-analyses
- www.update-software.com/publications/cochrane – The Cochrane Collaboration collects regularly updated systematic reviews of medical literature

BIBLIOGRAPHY

BOOKS

Ashton R, Leppard B 2005 Differential diagnosis in dermatology, 3rd edn. Radcliffe, Abingdon
A welcome new edition which adds in advice about management. A good book if you like an algorithm-based approach to diagnosis.

Burns T, Breathnach S, Cox N et al 2004 Rook's textbook of dermatology, 7th edn. Blackwell Science, Oxford
All of dermatology is in these four volumes, up to date and well illustrated.

Bolognia JL, Jorizzo JL, Rapini RP 2003 Dermatology. Mosby, Edinburgh
In addition to encyclopaedic information on skin disorders, this book is also available as an on-line resource, with all the illustrations from the book available as downloads onto PowerPoint.

Buxton PK 2005 ABC of dermatology, 4th edn. BMJ, London
A concise overview of the essentials of dermatology.

Gawkrodger DJ 1997 An illustrated colour text, 2nd edn. Churchill Livingstone, Edinburgh
If you ever read a dermatology text as a student, this is a good introduction.

Hunter J, Savin J, Dahl M 2002 Clinical dermatology, 3rd edn. Blackwell Science, Oxford
Good basic textbook, easy to read and interspersed with down to earth learning points.

ARTICLES FROM JOURNALS

Allan SJ, Kavanagh GM, Herd RM, Savin JA 2004 The effect of inositol supplements on the psoriasis of patients taking lithium: a randomized, placebo-controlled trial. BJD 150(5):966–969

Ashcroft DM, Li Wan Po A, Williams HC et al 2000 Systematic review of comparative efficacy and tolerability of calcipotriol in treating chronic plaque psoriasis. BMJ 320:963–967

Ashcroft DM, Dimmock P, Garside R et al 2005 Efficacy and tolerability of topical pimecrolimus and tacrolimus in the treatment of atopic dermatitis: meta analysis of randomised controlled trials. BMJ 330:516–522

Atherton DJ 2003 Topical corticosteroids in atopic dermatitis. BMJ 327:942–943

Barnetson RStC, Rogers M 2002 Childhood atopic eczema. BMJ 324:1376–1379

Boehncke W-H 2003 Immunomodulating drugs for psoriasis. BMJ 327:634–635

Charman C 1999 Clinical evidence: atopic eczema. BMJ 318:1600–1604

Fry A, Verne J 2003 Preventing skin cancer. BMJ 326:114–115

Hoare C, Li Wan Po A, Williams H 2000 Systematic review of treatments for atopic eczema. Health and Technology Assessment 4(37):1–191

Thomas KS, Armstrong S, Avery A et al 2002 Randomized controlled trial of short bursts of a potent topical corticosteroid versus prolonged use of a mild preparation for children with mild or moderate atopic eczema. BMJ 324:763

BRITISH JOURNAL OF DERMATOLOGY (BJD) GUIDELINES

Cox NH, Eady DJ, Morton CA 1999 Guidelines for management of Bowen's disease. BJD 141:633–641

Grattan C, Powell S, Humphreys F 2001 Guidelines for the management of urticaria and angioedema. BJD 144:708–714

Higgins EM, Fuller IC, Smith CH 2000 Guidelines for management of tinea capitis. BJD 143:53–58

MacDonald Hull SP, Wood ML, Hutchinson PE et al 2003 Guidelines for the management of alopecia areata. BJD 149:692–699

Motley R, Kersey P, Lawrence C 2002 Multiprofessional guidelines for the management of the patient with primary cutaneous squamous cell carcinoma. BJD 146:18–25

Roberts DLL, Anstey AV, Barlow RJ et al 2002 UK guidelines for the management of cutaneous melanoma. BJD 146:7–17

Roberts DT, Taylor WD, Boyle J 2003 Guidelines for the treatment of onychomycosis. BJD 148:402–410

Sterling JC, Handfield Jones S, Hudson PM 2001 Guidelines for the management of cutaneous warts. BJD 144:4–11

Telfer NR, Colver GB, Bowers PW 1999 Guidelines for the management of basal cell carcinoma. BJD 141:415–423

Wojnarowska F, Kirtschig G, Highet AS et al 2002 Guidelines for the management of bullous pemphigoid. BJD 147:214–221

DRUG AND THERAPEUTICS BULLETIN

2000 Compression therapy for venous ulcers. Drug and Therapeutics Bulletin (38) April

2002 Managing solar keratoses. Drug and Therapeutics Bulletin (40) May

2002 The management of sciatica. Drug and Therapeutics Bulletin (40) June

2002 Getting rid of athlete's foot. Drug and Therapeutics Bulletin (40) July

2002 Topical tacrolimus – a role in atopic dermatitis? Drug and Therapeutics Bulletin (40) October

2003 Topical steroids for atopic dermatitis in primary care. Drug and Therapeutics Bulletin (41) January

2003 Pimecrolimus cream for atopic dermatitis. Drug and Therapeutics Bulletin (41) May

2003 Acne, isotretinoin and depression. Drug and Therapeutics Bulletin (41) October

2004 Management of Bowen's disease of the skin. Drug and Therapeutics Bulletin (42) February

2004 Laser treatment for skin problems. Drug and Therapeutics Bulletin (42) October

2005 Probiotics for skin diseases. Drug and Therapeutics Bulletin (43) January

ELECTRONIC SOURCES

Cochrane collaboration reviews – excellent source of evidence-based reviews. Available: www.cochrane.org/reviews/index.htm

■ Antihistamines for atopic eczema
■ Chinese herbal medicine for atopic eczema
■ Combined oral contraceptive pills for treatment of acne
■ Complementary therapies for acne
■ Compression for preventing recurrence of venous ulcers
■ Compression for venous leg ulcers
■ Dressings and topical agents for leg ulcers
■ Dressings for venous ulcers
■ Interventions for active keratoses
■ Interventions for alopecia areata
■ Interventions for basal cell carcinoma of the skin
■ Interventions for bullous pemphigoid
■ Interventions for cellulitis and erysipelas
■ Interventions for chronic palmoplantar pustular psoriasis
■ Interventions for guttate psoriasis
■ Interventions for hand eczema
■ Interventions for impetigo
■ Interventions for photodamaged skin
■ Interventions for polymorphic light eruption
■ Interventions for rosacea

- Interventions to reduce Staphylococcus aureus for atopic eczema
- Laser resurfacing for facial acne scars
- Local treatments for cutaneous warts
- Maternal antigen avoidance during pregnancy and/or lactation for preventing or treating atopic disease in the child
- Minocycline for acne vulgaris: efficacy and safety
- Oral isotretinoin for acne
- Oral treatments for fungal infections of skin on the foot
- Physical treatments for non-complicated chronic venous insufficiency
- Soy formula for prevention of allergy and food intolerance in infants
- Systemic antifungal therapy for tinea capitis in children
- Topical treatments for chronic plaque psoriasis
- Topical treatments for fungal infections of the skin and nails of the foot

LIST OF PATIENT QUESTIONS

INDEX

Notes: page numbers in **bold** refer to boxes, figures and tables

A